DASA

(Dynamic Application of Spiritual Awareness)

Adym Dantz

ISBN 979-8-89130-030-9 (paperback)
ISBN 979-8-89130-031-6 (digital)

Copyright © 2024 by Adym Dantz

All rights reserved. No part of this publication may be reproduced, distributed, or transmitted in any form or by any means, including photocopying, recording, or other electronic or mechanical methods without the prior written permission of the publisher. For permission requests, solicit the publisher via the address below.

Christian Faith Publishing
832 Park Avenue
Meadville, PA 16335
www.christianfaithpublishing.com

Printed in the United States of America

To my children: Angel, Genesis, Moses, Sadoc, Jerusalem, Asiale, Divine, and Velvet.

Contents

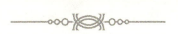

Acknowledgments vii
Introduction ix

Chapter 1:   The Breath 1
Chapter 2:   Dynamics of DASA 8
Chapter 3:   Correct Breathing 15
Chapter 4:   DASA at Work 26
Chapter 5:   Connecting Scriptures 34
Chapter 6:   Abandoned 48
Chapter 7:   The Hated Jew 52
Chapter 8:   The Godhead 57
Chapter 9:   Food from the Godhead 73
Chapter 10: Significance of Christ 94
Chapter 11: The Gospel Truth 98
Chapter 12: Right Side or Left Side 111
Chapter 13: The End-Times 117

Conclusion 123

Acknowledgments

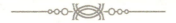

My literary agent, Kimberly Schwandt, who totally surprised me with the acceptance of my Holy Spirit–inspired work, receives my first acknowledgment. Of course, I also acknowledge my publication specialist, Ariel Jordan, as she was my liaison, practically "holding my hand" while guiding me through the entire process from pre-editing to publication.

Special thanks go to the Christian Faith Publishing staff responsible for weaving together all the parts necessary to form this work into a credible source of spiritual information, as well as making it aesthetically pleasing to the reader.

James A. McKenzie's significant contribution to this work was absolutely invaluable, and I greatly praise and thank Almighty Jesus Christ (Revelation 1:8) for using my beloved brother as the agent I worked through to jump-start this project and keep it going. My brother-in-Christ, Patrick Cannavan, deserves acknowledgment for kindly and unselfishly perusing some chapters of this work and offering valued suggestions. And also to Brother Solo, who worked in the meat processing industry and provided firsthand information on the sheer grossness of "meat byproducts."

Introduction

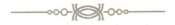

DASA is a Holy Spirit–inspired program of this award-winning author, father of eight children, and former competitor in kung fu tournaments. As his blessing to you, this highly regarded work will arm you with the necessary *tools* to lessen the effects of stress-inducing negative emotions while greatly enhancing spiritual awareness. This level of understanding grants you the ability to apply this method dynamically (i.e., moment by moment, in every phase of life, in every situation). Your spirit, soul, and body are positively impacted as the principles of the gospel of Christ are infused into your lifestyle.

Bear in mind, however, that physical emotions have no bearing on your engagement and subsequent success in reaching the level of perpetual DASA mode. At this level, the principles of God's word of truth will be intrinsically applied to all you may think or speak. DASA is indeed a comprehensive program that guides you to live a complete lifestyle consistent with God's will (Galatians 5:25). Moreover, you should experience a quality, physical equanimity as a new life is spiritually *breathed* into you so that your behavior, actions, and service to Almighty God will be effective, spiritually rewarding, and positively impact your surrounding society and even have lasting significance.

It is worth repeating, and I emphatically express to you that your physical emotions have absolutely zero effect within the practice and usage of DASA. The only modality you will operate in is the realm of faith, which, in all actuality, is a loving gift from the Father of lights (James 1:17). With Proverbs 3:5 in mind, you will lean on His word of truth in Romans 3:30 and 4:16 to help you understand

God-given faith. For without it, you will never advance to perpetual *DASA mode and fulfill the requirements* God purposed for you (Hebrews 11:6). To make it even more clear, faith is the confidence that what we hope for will actually be manifested by the Father of all creation, in whom we place our trust; it gives us assurance about the things we cannot yet see (Hebrews 11:1).

Accompanying the intrinsic requirement of faith given to us through God's grace, there are physical gifts innate to us, consistent with the Godhead's tripartite nature; they are as follows: air, water, and food. Both the water and the food were supplied at "the creation" or "in the beginning" (Genesis 1:1, 11). The air (i.e., our breath), however, was personal when the Lord Himself breathed His holy breath directly into our lungs through our nostrils—holy CPR perhaps? Just contemplate that. The invisible substance we inhale/exhale billions of times during our lifespan is the Lord's holy breath. Interestingly, He called for us to be holy even before He created us (Ephesians 1:4). Essentially, we were created by the Godhead using a three-stage process.

1. He formed our spirit (Zechariah 12:1).
2. He scooped up elements of the earth (i.e., a pile of dirt, molded it into a particular shape—human, and infused it with the spirit, that is, the real you He formed) (Genesis 1:26–27).
3. He gave vitality to that "pile of dirt"—our terrestrial body—by breathing His holy breath into it (Genesis 2:7).

Just as the Godhead used a three-stage process in our creation, you will, in effect, utilize a three-stage process in the practice of DASA:

1. Learn to appreciate and respect the value of this holy breath of God, which is on loan to us temporarily. This is achieved by breathing correctly and fully to calm and relax your mind and body.

DASA (DYNAMIC APPLICATION OF SPIRITUAL AWARENESS)

2. Initiate DASA in that tranquil state, resulting in a vibrant, joyous way to do the works God purposed for you (Ephesians 2:10).
3. Take care of ourselves with both spiritual nutrition (Matthew 4:4) and proper nutritional supplementation until we ultimately are changed (i.e., receive our new BBG—body by God) (1 Corinthians 15:51–52; 2 Corinthians 5:1).

Chapter 1

The Breath

The Godhead, identified by the statement, "Let Us… Our image… like Us," in Genesis 1:26, created our lungs for a specific purpose. That purpose is to draw in a quantity of air to oxygenate the entire body, from the brain to the feet, and expel carbon dioxide (i.e., the air you inhale is not the same as what your lungs exhale). Moreover, according to one's body size, lungs are proportionally designed and created exclusively for each individual human body type. Hence, the full capacity of your lungs can supply your body with the appropriate quantity of air necessary for the healthy integrity of both internal organs and external body members.

Now here is where one of the main problems lies that is both associated with and negatively impacts one's emotions; it is shallow breathing. What that implies is you are not inhaling, with every single breath, the quantity of air the Godhead created your lungs for. If it were not for the inbuilt function of yawning and sighing, which forces a sufficient quantity of air to full lung capacity throughout each day, perhaps multitudes of people would keel over and expire simply from a lack of oxygen due to shallow breathing, or what I call *lazy breathing*.

Whether the so-called professionals choose to admit it or not, I am fully convinced that by not taking *whole breaths*, that is, each and every breath expands the lungs to full capacity, you are cheating your body of much of its daily requirement of this invisible nutrient called air. Various body cells operate erratically, function poorly, or simply die without oxygen. When this happens, and especially when it is sustained over a long period of time, your body becomes vulnerable to a host of health issues related to the interference of normal operations, including emotional instability. Unfortunately, this is where the pharmaceutical industry, in association with the majority of allopathic doctors (MDs), has a "field day" reaping a financial windfall by plying people with more unnecessary, useless, negative side effect–producing meds than wrinkles in old people; they even have drugs for wrinkles.

It is unfortunately a sad reality that all too many people take breathing, like so many other of the Godhead's wonderful gifts to us, for granted and do not use it to its full potential. And just why is that? Well, for the most part, much of it may be attributable to emotions. People tend to lean heavily on their own emotions in an attempt to pacify themselves. But they quickly learn that physical emotions are not tenable, which compels them to seek some type of inanimate object to gaze at, touch, rub, or manipulate with their fingers, or they overindulge in eating nonnutritious snacks and drinks, or even more destructively, their crutch is that of abusing one or more habit-forming, toxic, liquid, or chemical drug. So in addition to already breathing lazily, people nonchalantly poison God's marvelous, highest, and last creation—the human (Genesis 1:26). Compounded, all these negative "forces" trigger the body's built-in protective mechanisms to operate in perpetual overdrive until, boom! The resiliency of the internal and/or external body components is compromised, and adverse health becomes your antagonist and constant reminder of your inadequacy, mortality, and absolute inability to solve your life problems either through your own means or via myriad humanistic measures. And for that, the Godhead made something so very plain and clear to you in Proverbs 3:5–8.

Improper Breathing

As already mentioned, lazy breathing is not conducive to thriving health. In association with your emotions, it could change you

DASA (DYNAMIC APPLICATION OF SPIRITUAL AWARENESS)

into a fitful, nerve-racking ball of anxiety, depression, despair, discouragement, hypertension, and worry because your body's central processing unit (the brain) is not being adequately and consistently supplied with the oxygen necessary to support the activity of the billions of cells your brain perpetually engages in to properly regulate these negative emotions. Every single second, your body is busy both creating and destroying a portion of the succession of multiple billions of cells as they traverse their internal perimeters.

Basically, there are two ways you short your lungs of sufficient air supply:

1. You take very small breaths during your normal, daily breathing.
2. You lift your chest—maybe shoulders too—when you think you are taking a deep breath.

Another negative result of shorting your lungs of the required amount of oxygen is becoming sleepy at some of the most inappropriate times: during a church sermon, an important business meeting, a school classroom lecture, at your computer on the job, and one of the most deadly, while driving a vehicle on the freeway, other roads, or even city streets. Thousands of lives have been and are still being lost resulting from this unnecessary yet avoidable evil.

As you live, move, and breathe, there is a 24-7 flowing and ebbing of body cells from head to toe which churns ceaselessly until shortly after your final breath of life. Actually, an amazing thing begins to occur at that point. The body reverses its course and begins consuming itself (i.e., decomposing) as it returns to the elements of the earth.

Breathing improperly (shallow or lazy breathing) dramatically shortens the lifespan of a body cell in addition to it becoming dysfunctional. And when a cell cannot do what its function requires, other cells are forced to carry its load while attempting to continue their own operations. Multiplied many times over, this puts undue stress on the entire system, dragging it down. When this happens with something as vital as the immune system, your body is unable to keep up with and fight off the incessant invasion of hundreds of various types of foreigners (bacteria, viruses, and parasites) bombarding you through your nostrils, mouth, and skin. Think about it for a while; all this agony simply because you are too lazy to do one thing—breathe properly!

To add insult to injury is the misapplied way people are taught to take in a deep breath. When you are asked to take a deep breath, you probably breathe in while lifting your chest, shoulders, and chin. Perhaps unknowingly, you have just shorted hundreds of thousands of cells of the oxygen necessary to carry out their intended purpose. And most allopathic doctors (MD) don't even bother to correct you; many of them couldn't care less, as they are all too eager to offload their latest pharmaceutical drug on you, draining your wallet.

Bear this in mind; when you lift your chest/shoulders/head area to suck in a deep breath, you cut off a significant portion of air that should be flowing into the bottom of the lungs first, expanding there, then the air fills the lungs from bottom to top. It is a shame, but an unfortunate reality, that the ones you entrust your health to shortchange you in two ways: your health and your wallet. It has happened for millennia (Mark 5:25–26).

Time for a Change

Have you ever heard or used the phrase "It's time to breathe new life into it"? Well, if you are just tired of being "sick and tired," and having your emotions wreak havoc on your psyche and physicality, DASA, *with the Word of God* as its foundation, will help you learn to breathe new *life* into your internal body, adding and supporting vibrant physical/mental health, while God's refreshing word of truth pours nourishment and vitality into your malnourished spiritual body. In the dynamic application of spiritual awareness, you feel the air flowing through your nose and into your lungs to nourish your body; that is, by feeling, you know the air is going in. With the Scriptures, you sense the word of God flowing through your eyes and into your soul to nourish your spirit; that is, by faith, you know the word is being planted within. DASA relaxes your mind, revital-

DASA (DYNAMIC APPLICATION OF SPIRITUAL AWARENESS)

izes your body, and positively impacts and stabilizes your emotions. The word of God, with no attachment to your human emotions, strengthens your spirit by the Holy Spirit (2 Corinthians 5:15). Together, DASA and the word of God help you engage in the work of God without being thwarted by negative emotions and allow you to worship Him in spirit and truth, not in superficial emotional ecstasy (John 4:24).

Following are two excellent scriptural examples of DASA when it is put into operation, and when people allow circumstances to frazzle their emotions; one is taken from the Old Testament, the other from the New:

Elijah, a prophet sent by God (1 Kings 18:1), was on the "Most Wanted" poster of an exploitative king, as mentioned in 1 Kings 18:10. Nevertheless, secure in DASA mode, Elijah remained undaunted. He went head-to-head against the king and 850 men who were a combination of the king and his wife's false prophets. Elijah defeated them all with relative ease, made them feel like fools, and then killed them all in the Kishon Valley with a spectacular defeat. Then to top that off, Elijah, still in DASA mode, outran the king's horses for seventeen miles from Mt. Carmel to the city of Jezreel to escape the fast-approaching thunderstorm. Let me see you try to outrun even a pony.

Now like so many others, Elijah allowed his physical emotions to interfere with his dynamic application of spiritual awareness, as shown when he became deathly afraid of and intimidated by the threat of the king's wife: "May the gods strike me and even kill me if by this time tomorrow I have not killed you as you killed them." Emotionally, he was so afraid that he ran for his life—for forty days and forty nights. He went all the way to Mt. Sinai, about two hundred miles away. All during that time, (1) he threw a pity party; (2) he experienced anxiety, depression, loneliness, and worry; and (3) he became suicidal. You may read about it all in 1 Kings chapters 18–19.

About 850 years later, we find another man, a ragtag, hardworking, married fisherman, probably with minimal education, from a small Galilean town named Bethsaida. Along with eleven others, he was chosen by God to become an apostle of Jesus the Messiah (Luke

5

6:12–16). Outspoken and impulsive, he became the natural leader of the group who would be mentored by the Messiah and experience innumerable, unprecedented events (miracles) he thought only happened with ancient ancestors like Enoch, Noah, Moses, and the prophets.

Somewhere in the middle of the Sea of Galilee, as the local people called this huge lake, about 3:00 a.m., the boat the apostles were in got caught in a strong wind, and they struggled, rowing against the rough waves. All of a sudden, they thought they saw a ghost and, like in some late-night horror show, they screamed in terror. But then, a familiar voice came from what they thought was a ghost walking on the *sea*. Vernacularly speaking, the "supposed ghost" said, "Hey, relax, fellas. It's Me."

Of all people, it was the impulsive one, whom Jesus named Peter, who spoke up and started thinking in DASA mode after hearing his Master's voice. Peter, with his eyes intently focused on Jesus instead of the strong wind and heavy waves, requested permission to walk on the sea toward Jesus. On His approval, Peter, now in full DASA mode, while focusing on Jesus, stepped out of the boat and actually walked on the water out in the middle of the sea. You can accomplish impossible odds with Christ (Philippians 4:13).

Again, as too many believers do, this man, this chosen one, like Elijah had done about eight centuries prior, began looking around him at the circumstances (strong wind, dashing waves), whereas Peter allowed his human emotions to veto his DASA, and the inevitable happened; he began to sink. This all takes place in Matthew 14:22–32.

So as you should have surmised from those two of hundreds of scriptural examples, DASA is not like a static, frozen-in-time-space picture or photo; it is not a do-it-one-time thing. It is when you dynamically (continuously) apply the awareness of your spirit to the reality and truth of the word of God on a daily, 24-7 basis. I think you might need to read that sentence over again to fully comprehend what I am saying to you. In fact, perhaps you should highlight it with a marker and come back to it often until it is crystal clear to you. Get with someone else and ask him/her their opinion, and discuss it.

DASA (DYNAMIC APPLICATION OF SPIRITUAL AWARENESS)

About as easily as I can break it down for you is by going back to our two main characters, Elijah and Peter. On each occasion, a directive was spoken by the Lord. With Elijah, He said, "Go..." (1 Kings 18:1). With Peter, He said, "Come..." (Matthew 14:29). So coupled with the gift of faith that God supplies to His true believers, they ignored what their emotions were shouting to them about the circumstances, and instead, they used DASA to home in on the directive (the word of God) and each one was able to overcome overwhelming odds (also ref. Proverb 3:5–6).

Chapter 2

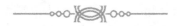

Dynamics of DASA

As you begin to wonder more and more about the DASA method, be advised that it is not a tangible object you touch or gaze upon with your physical eyes. Neither do you venture into some trancelike state of mind, chanting or murmuring monotone sounds on and on, as you sit in a certain position. There are no special hats, clothing, shoes, rugs, figurines (dolls), or other paraphernalia you need to be involved in the practice of DASA. To clarify, there is no specific way to sit; you may stand, sit, kneel, stoop, squat, or even crawl if that's your thing; you might not want to do that in public, though, as they might take you away in a straitjacket.

What's more, DASA is not a certain routine you dedicate a set amount of time to, several days a week like other human endeavors; it is not a temporary trend, hobby, fad, something done for enjoyment from time to time, nor necessarily team-oriented, though discussion of its specifics may be of some benefit.

As a reminder, DASA assists greatly in helping you disengage from your human, negative emotions, and tune in, instead, to the spiritual wisdom and understanding God desires to give you. And while in this perpetual mode, you apply the principles of the word of God to your total lifestyle in a way that will truly honor the God you claim to believe in (Romans 12:1). Moreover, this mindset will guide you into worshiping God, not by manmade religious rituals,

DASA (DYNAMIC APPLICATION OF SPIRITUAL AWARENESS)

candles, incense, and other useless religiosity, but by the Almighty's way (John 4:24).

Dynamic application of spiritual awareness is an intrinsic quality within you that has been hindered by two main antagonists: (1) Satan—1 Peter 5:8; (2) Yourself—James 1:14. You see, Satan is a powerful, evil spiritual being you cannot fight against physically. He enters you to influence you from within (John 13:27; Ephesians 6:12). And if that wasn't already bad enough, you make it worse with your own evil thoughts (Matthew 15:19). It is obvious that people do not realize how serious this is; they take it as some type of joke. But this is no game. Giving in to your passionate desires and entertaining your evil thoughts actually separate you from God and make you His enemy (Colossians 1:21). And to show you how serious it is, read Philippians 3:18 and James 4:4. Do you really want to keep playing around like that and fall into the judgment of the living God who is a consuming fire (Hebrews 10:31; 12:29)? Go ahead and continue in your "fun" now, but you will pay later. Guess what God will do to His enemies? Read Isaiah 3:9 and 59:18.

Again, DASA cannot become available to you through your emotions. It is a real, but invisible quality that you tap into with nothing but sheer, unadulterated faith that comes from God Himself (Matthew 4:4; Romans 10:17). DASA is exclusive to the word of God because, in His marvelous word, your eyes will be opened to what spiritual awareness is. All I am doing, as an ambassador for Christ, is coaching you on how to apply the principles of this word of truth in *real time*. Before continuing on, it is important to know the three main ingredients that are inseparable: the word of God, DASA, and faith. You simply cannot have one without the other. Romans 10:17 may also be viewed in this manner. God develops faith within you as you begin to pay attention (hearing, intently listening, or reading with interest) to His word, where you will learn about spiritual awareness. So therefore, all three are contained within the other like wetness is contained in water; you cannot separate the wet from the water. You must continue to believe this truth and stand firm (Colossians 1:23).

The reason why breathing plays a role in DASA is because of what I so emphatically explained to you in chapter 1; it helps your body to be fully oxygen-nourished from head to toe and is instrumental in maintaining a calm, relaxed demeanor as it keeps your emotions in check. While living in this earthly domain, our spirits operate through this earthly body. Our human emotions have a tendency to continuously tug at this body to pull it downward toward a worldly lifestyle. That is why the dynamic (real-time) application (take-now-action) of spiritual awareness (perceiving your inner being) should be to your spirit, what the heart is to the body—nonstop pumping action. And I want to drill into you that faith is the key here, not your emotions. By the faith God has given us (Romans 12:3), you need to struggle against your flesh and depend on God's supernatural power working in you (Colossians 1:29).

I am going to keep reminding you of that first word in DASA— *dynamic*. It can also relate to something or someone living. That is, you are dynamic (living), while a comatose person is not. Does that adverb (dynamic) have any significance to you now? Going overboard in explaining this does not bother me. I sincerely want you to fully grasp this so that when you feel you are ready to engage in DASA, you will not allow negative emotions to compel you to look around for an "off switch" during hard times, pressure, unexpected circumstances, tribulations, or other situations that may potentially have a negative impact.

With faith being key, God gives it freely, which helps you to help Him, help you help Him. Your "always on" DASA-mode is tuned into God's power working in you. As you learn to dwell in and live your lifestyle in this mode, the Lord will reveal to you things that you were previously blind to (2 Corinthians 4:4). To spur you on, here is something that should cause you to take in a deep breath: That power of God in you is dynamic; it is living, but it is not a "living energy" as some false religions will try to make you believe. That power of God in you is a Person, and that Person is none other than Christ Jesus Himself. DASA will reveal to you through the word of God that our Savior is both the power of God and the wisdom of God (1 Corinthians 1:24). That is one of the dynamics of DASA.

DASA (DYNAMIC APPLICATION OF SPIRITUAL AWARENESS)

Mystery Revealed

If you are troubled by what must have been a shocking revelation to you, I can understand that. Being the loving God that He is, full of truth and grace, God's patience will overlook your probable temporary hesitant position as He gently guides you in His truth.

Unlike many of the so-called *secret* societies or organizations spreading out across planet Earth, having secret codes, handshakes, verbal expressions, emblems, or such, Almighty God, the creator of everything that exists, is not prone to that sort of worldliness. His ways are beyond that (Isaiah 55:8–9). But despite that heavenly loftiness, He bridged the gap through Jesus, who is the Messiah (Christ). This is the only way the holy God of the universe connects with this sinful world. And through God's power (i.e., through Jesus), God actually wants us to understand His mystery plan that was not yet revealed to the Old Testament prophets (1 Peter 1:10–11).

Operating in the mode of dynamically applying your spiritual awareness to your daily lifestyle will develop within you a desire to personally connect with God in a much stronger and deeper way. Christ is God's mystery plan. I repeat: the mystery plan of God is in the form of a Person. God took to bridge the gap between sinful humanity and the perfect, holy One He is by clothing Himself in a human body so that He could speak with us face-to-face, man-to-man, up close and personal. In DASA mode, it will help you comprehend the truth of God's word that when you look at (or believe in) Jesus, you see God, and God speaks through Jesus all that He wants us to know (John 12:45, 49). Being in DASA mode 24-7 will both improve and increase, as well as strengthen, your spiritual awareness, your study of God's word, your prayers (communication) to Him; your singing of praise songs will be more meaningful, and you will know the real value of worshiping Him in spirit and truth (John 4:24).

When a mystery is kept secret, people give way to opinions, conjecture, half-truths, misinformation, and silly myths. But through Christ, God has made known the secret, and now all the treasures of wisdom and knowledge are available to you (Colossians 2:3). To be absolutely and brutally honest, the world's view of Christ is in the first sentence of this paragraph. And 95 percent of what you see and hear on television and radio on the world's holidays, especially so-called Easter and Christmas, is mass-produced, world-class junk. Instead, being in DASA mode will assure you that Christ lives in you (Romans 8:10); you are clothed in Him (Romans 13:14). He makes His home in you (Ephesians 3:17).

The Clue

DASA will enlighten you regarding the clues to the *hidden* secrets or *mysteries* contained in the word of God. The more interest you show and the more time you invest in His word of truth, Jesus will reveal greater truths to you. The entire word of God is replete with clues that connect to, corroborate, or substantiate one another. Here is an example to give you an idea. Once I seriously submitted my life to Christ, invested quality time in studying the Scriptures every single day for several hours a day, and became truly interested in the lives of the various biblical characters, the Lord began helping me retain information about certain events, places, names of people, and other happenings.

As I was studying the book of Colossians again for the umpteenth time, when I was pondering 1:15 trying to understand the deeper meaning of it, my spiritual thought reflected on when Philip very bluntly let Jesus know that he and the other apostles wanted to actually see the Father, whose voice they heard from heaven (Luke 9:35; John 12:28). And very straightforwardly, Jesus let Philip know that Jesus Himself was the Father (John 14:8–9). Then I also remembered another Scripture I had studied several times over a few years. It was Colossians 2:9, saying how all the fullness of the Godhead lived in Christ. When the Holy Spirit revealed to me that Jesus is the Father through those three Scripture clues (John 14:8–9; Colossians 1:15; 2:9), I was awestruck.

Having even more enthusiasm for "secrets" to be revealed to me, I made a stern decision not to be the lukewarm, flimsy, average "Christian" that so many people masquerade as. To me, it was all or

DASA (DYNAMIC APPLICATION OF SPIRITUAL AWARENESS)

nothing. I opted for all, made it a point to be a Luke 9:23 Christ-follower, and I believed in God and took decisive action on Proverbs 3:9 and 19:17, along with Malachi 3:10. Since then, the Lord has been true to His word, and I am blessed beyond my wildest expectations. What's even better than the physical, material blessings I enjoy is who and what God made me to be. Here is what I am and have in Christ:

- an actual son of God (Romans 8:16)
- an heir (Galatians 4:7)
- a guaranteed inheritance (Ephesians 1:14; 1 Peter 1:4)
- heavenly citizenship (Philippians 3:20; Colossians 3:1–3)
- a first-class, one-way ticket reservation (1 Thessalonians 4:16–17)

I trust God 1 million percent (Numbers 23:19; Proverbs 3:5; and Hebrews 6:18), and I will joyfully do the work(s) He has assigned me to do during my sojourn here on Earth as I wait for His rock-solid, iron-clad promises (John 14:1–3; 1 Corinthians 2:9). Additionally, I will continue to be studious in the word of truth so I may be of service to everyone the Lord gives me the privilege of serving, and the opportunity to share this gospel with.

For thousands of years, those who truly believe, reverence, obey, and serve God have been mocked, scorned, hated, and persecuted by the masses of humanity. It does not bother me in the least; Jesus said for us to have no fear of humans, and that, like Him, we will suffer persecution (Luke 12:4; John 15:18, 20). And here we are in the technologically advanced, digital age with today's skeptics and naysayers ridiculing me and saying I am trusting in a pie-in-the-sky pipe dream.

Way too many of my brothers and sisters who truly love the Lord and desire deep in their hearts to be obedient to the Lord are rankled by their emotions, as well as being spiritually challenged. You are not aware that as you open God's word, there are clues all around you. By simply dabbling in the word of God, instead of taking it as seriously as you take air, water, and food, you will remain on the level that the Apostle Paul had to admonish saints about (1 Corinthians 3:1–2; Hebrews 5:11–14).

Saints, with the downhill slide of society pulling you downward toward destruction by their new-fangled words and terms (i.e., *politically correct, identity politics, "smash heteronormativity," gender-affirming care, wokeness, transgender, critical race theory, cancel culture*, and many other leftist rhetoric), you cannot sit by in your quagmire of mediocrity and spiritual lethargy, or Satan will gore you like a maniacal Wisconsin bull. So to whet a spiritual appetite in you so that you will be armed with some word of God ammunition in your transitioning to DASA, get warmed up with these connecting Scriptural clues:

- You belong to God because He not only purchased you, but He also paid a ransom for you (1 Corinthians 6:20; 1 Peter 1:18–19).
- Satan has no power over the Spirit of Christ (John 12:31); the Spirit of Christ is in you (Romans 8:9); and the Spirit of Christ in you is greater than the spirit of Satan in this world (1 John 4:4).
- Your stand against the spirit of Satan is your faith (Ephesians 6:16); be strong in Christ, resist the devil, and he will flee from you (James 4:7; 1 Peter 5:9).

Snack on those for a while until you are firmly convinced that this is some vital, wholesome, spiritually delicious nutrition that will jump-start you.

Chapter 3

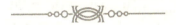

Correct Breathing

In chapter 1, you gained some insight about your breath. No, I'm not talking about that smelly halitosis that makes you want to dive off the bed away from your spouse in the mornings. I'm talking about how you inhale that vital, invisible substance so desperately needed for the totality of your body, and to sustain the operating integrity of internal components: brain, heart, immune system, cardiovascular system, kidneys, liver, spleen, and others that work cohesively supporting every single movement, even the tiniest movements such as the blink of your eyes.

As the Godhead created us, He designed two large airbag-type components in our upper abdominal cavity with many string-like attachments (passageways) connecting to the body. What the Godhead did in Genesis 2:7 caused airflow through those numerous, thin, flexibly soft tubes that carried God's breath of life throughout this "body by God."

Because of that, the apostle's statement in Acts 17:28 should be more meaningful to you; it is the very breath of Almighty God that sustains us. Think long and serious about that. The breath you inhale hundreds of times on a daily basis is not yours; it belongs to the Godhead, who is the *Us* in Genesis 1:26. And it is only on loan to you. He can take it away at His choosing (Deuteronomy 32:39). So it is in your best interest to take full advantage and use those two airbags (lungs) to full capacity to preclude brain cells and other cells from being created with severely limited functioning and dying prematurely.

You were enlightened earlier, in "the Clue," of the Godhead's dual nature as the Father and Jesus. However, He (the Godhead) is actually a tripartite Entity, which many clues in Scripture reveal in DASA mode. But I will toss this in because it slightly relates to the context of this breathing topic. Who is the Godhead? He is the Father (Deuteronomy 32:6), He is the Word (John 1:1), and He is the Holy Spirit (Galatians 4:6; Ephesians 4:4). And my prayer for you is this: May His power within you motivate you to use the faith He granted to you in continuously and successfully applying spiritual awareness dynamically to every phase of your lifestyle. I mentioned that to show you how the Godhead made our physical existence contingent upon a tripartite action: breathing, drinking, and eating. In fact, the nature of the Godhead is stamped literally upon the entire universe. But, sticking with the topic of this discussion, air takes precedence over water and food; air is the highest priority.

With every breath you inhale, it should be a reminder of how thankful you should be to God for lending His breath to you. And mark my word, it is only a matter of time before it (your breath on loan) becomes due. So do not skimp on your breathing; breathe each and every inhalation to the full capacity of your lungs, as God designed them to hold. Not only will you derive exponential benefits healthwise for doing so, but you will also be honoring God as He observes you make full use of His ingeniously complex design (Proverbs 15:3; 1 Peter 3:12). As for smoking, no need for me to go into much detail on that, as an incredible mountain of facts speaks for themselves. Smoking is a filthy, habit-forming activity that poisons our God-created lungs, is a way of committing slow suicide, shows that you hate your own body, dishonors God, and shows contempt and total disrespect for His holy temple (1 Corinthians 3:16–17). With that said, DASA and smoking are contrary to each other. Nevertheless, DASA can help you quit that God-hating habit abruptly and totally, but only if you truly love God more (Matthew 22:37; Luke 9:23).

DASA (DYNAMIC APPLICATION OF SPIRITUAL AWARENESS)

Let's practice

In illustration A, you have two balloons. One shows the direction of airflow, while the other shows the results. Notice how the bottom of the balloon expands first. Then the upper portion begins expanding outward as the air rises. Pay particular attention to the fact that the incoming air does not expand first at the top of the balloon. By doing this yourself with an actual balloon, you might get a better idea and understanding.

Illustration A[1]

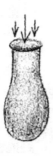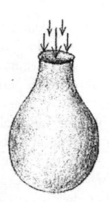

As the illustration clearly demonstrates, the air flows through the top—bypassing it—to reach the bottom, pushing it downward first before rising upward. Again, it is the air itself that is doing the work of filling and stretching the balloon from inside out, and in an upward direction. No other force is moving or lifting the balloon. Having that understanding should help you mentally picture how you should breathe.

Since there are obviously those who have no idea whatsoever what the lungs look like, illustration B provides that visual representation to help you mentally grasp this concept as well as physically feel this happening in real-time.

---

[1] https://i.pinimg.com/736x/77/69de8cb979ba68c1370F6fedc109a9.jpeg.

Illustration B[2]

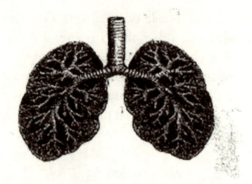

With the balloon as your guide, when you inhale, do not physically lift your chin, shoulders, and chest or pull in your belly. Just remain relaxed and direct your breath downward. When done in this way, you should both see and feel something happening. If you thought that your belly is expanding because you are pushing your breath down into it, you are absolutely wrong.

Directly under your lungs, between them and your stomach, is a type of muscle, stretching from left to right, called the diaphragm. As your breath travels down, expanding the bottom of your lungs, they press down on the diaphragm, which, in turn, presses down on top of the stomach, causing it to protrude outward. Of course, looking at this activity from outside the body makes it appear as though breath is going into the stomach. However, the stomach does not like air, just as the lungs do not like liquid or food particles. Swallow some air and see what happens; it will either come up front as a burp or go out back as a *bang*! And if even the smallest drop of liquid or tiniest food particle accidentally is inhaled into the windpipe, you will heave, gasp, retch, and cough roughly as your lungs violently protest.

I could be very profound in explaining the exemplary benefits of breath as I did in my previous award-winning book, but for the most part, all the information you need to be involved in DASA is

---

[2] https://i.pinimg.com/736x/77/69de8cb979ba68c1370F6fedc109a9.jpeg.

DASA (DYNAMIC APPLICATION OF SPIRITUAL AWARENESS)

above. The only thing you need to do now is to review all I have written above and actually do the breathing instead of just reading about it. Follow the steps below.

Breathing Steps

Because you have breathed lazily practically your entire life and have come to be comfortable with it, doing it correctly may be an inconvenience when starting out. It may not feel right. It may seem too challenging, and you may think that no one can breathe that way 24-7. And you are right. I do not disagree with you if that is the mindset you choose to adopt. I never argue with such negative opinions. As an ambassador for Christ, I simply instruct, demonstrate, and advise people with the compassion and love the Lord placed in me, hoping I can motivate them to push past the substandard worldly ways that cause complacency and imbalance in their lives.

For those ready to exit lazy breathing and "breathe new life" into that ol' body, begin by taking the next step.

Step 1:

The very first thing, good and pleasing to the Lord, you may want to do when you notice you are awake each morning—whether your eyes are closed or you open them as you are still prone—is to begin communicating with Him. Let Him know how appreciative you are of Him watching over and protecting you as you sleep. Thank Him for the new day He brought you into and, if you'd like to, tell Him about what you felt about a particular passage of Scripture you may have read, studied, or meditated on the previous night; sing a song of praise to Him from your heart (Psalm 7:17; Psalm 147:1). Smile once in a while as you are in this communication mode with the Lord. When you are done, whether you do it for a few minutes or an hour or more—because He should be first and foremost—then either as you are still lying there or after you have sat upright, close your eyes and start breathing correctly:

A. Take five to fifteen seconds to inhale (depending on your size).
B. Breathe out slowly until your tummy sinks in.
C. Repeat this without fail every morning for one week.
D. Start this practice with an easy five inhales/exhales daily.

Step 2:

If you succeeded in engaging in that breathing session each morning, it should pose no problem for you now. Here's what is next:

A. Take five to fifteen seconds to inhale. Check to ensure you are relaxed, not sucking in your stomach or lifting your chest.
B. Exhale easily, not quickly nor forcibly.
C. One set equals both A and B; do five sets.
D. Sometime during the afternoon, between twelve and three o'clock, take the time to engage in a round of five sets.
E. Do step D for one week straight; no excuses.

Step 3:

Be honest: did you engage in steps 1 and 2 over the past two weeks completely with no interruptions? If so, go ahead and communicate to the Lord how thankful you are. Also, you should be more comfortable breathing full breaths in the mornings and afternoons. If you want to take another week to engage in steps 1 and 2, by all means, go right ahead and enjoy yourself; there is no rush. But should you desire more challenge, then get with it.

A. Take five to fifteen seconds to inhale.
B. You may find that you can control the exhale much better by pursing your lips and exhaling through your mouth.
C. Do ten sets both in the mornings and afternoons for two weeks.

DASA (DYNAMIC APPLICATION OF SPIRITUAL AWARENESS)

Step 4:

One month has gone by as you have faithfully engaged in breathing practice. You should now notice the significant difference between your lazy breathing and correct breathing. Now having gone this far, why stop now? You are beginning something that results in manifold health benefits for you. In this, do you realize what you have done? You have taken a vested interest in an aspect of your life and health where the interest is exponentially compounded in terms of quality of life. You may not have noticed any significant changes, or perhaps you have noticed some slight differences. Every person is unique and experiences tolerances and changes quite differently from one person to the next. Now if you have made it this far, having fully engaged in steps 1 to 3, somewhere along the line here in step 4, you should begin to notice considerable results. Again, should you have the notion that you should spend more time on any of the previous steps, do not feel ashamed or believe you will be *left behind*, as it may be more beneficial in the long run. So stop here, do a 180° turn, and go back to engage in any step you feel most comfortable with. Everyone else, full speed ahead.

A. Take five to fifteen seconds to inflate your lungs.
B. Gently exhale, fully emptying your lungs.
C. Do ten sets. You will get the most benefit by moving as far away as possible from distractions like TV, radio, people gossiping, rap music, or any other loud, jarring distractions. By contrast, it may be more beneficial to play soft, soothing Christian praise music. Close your eyes and do not rush through; take your time.
D. Engage in step four three times daily—morning, noon, and night.
E. Practice this step daily for thirty days, with no excuses.

Congratulations! If, since you began practicing these controlled breathing sessions over the past nearly sixty days, you remained steadfast in it without missing a beat, heaven may be smiling down on you because you are seriously concerned about the high value of your lungs and the great benefits that may be derived from them when utilized the way God intended.

As a reminder, in addition to the many physical health benefits gained from engaging in this practice, it prepares you to operate in DASA mode no matter what the circumstances around you. Believe me! I know firsthand that engaging in this practice was no "stroll in the park." I have already been there, done that. But more than likely, you cannot deny the benefits you have now gained. And yours are not necessarily the same as another's.

Now here are some smart tips for your edification. You might not want to close your eyes if you are practicing this breathing in places like New York City's Central Park or Los Angeles' Pershing Square.

No problem, though, in a nice place like the Mall of Asia in Manila. I even performed a Heaven's Palm Tai Chi demonstration there to a large crowd of people previously. I look forward to traveling there again to converse with Christ-followers who are both practicing this controlled breathing and those who are effectively using DASA. Also, as I practiced in Davao City's Magsaysay Park, I noticed the group of Qigong (Chi-gung) practitioners there. When I return there, I'm hoping to find some DASA practitioners.

You are undoubtedly thinking, "Now what do I do?" That's a good question. And here is your good answer: you have now prepared yourself for step 5, the last step of instruction. It will be the most challenging for you to get prepared to operate 24-7 in DASA mode. When you are ready to make that move, however, and only you will know, you will discover that the outcome will be well worth the effort.

Before moving into step 5, let's do some checkups to ensure all is going well so that we do not continue with nor carry any incorrect practices that would jeopardize the integrity of ongoing training:

- As you perform the ten sets, both the inhale and exhale together equal one count (i.e., one set).

DASA (DYNAMIC APPLICATION OF SPIRITUAL AWARENESS)

- If you happen to be sharing practice with another individual, and that person is only five feet two inches tall and about eighty-five pounds, while you are a strapping six feet three inches, 280-pound behemoth, the differences in lung size will make the timing of the inhale/exhale quite different between each of you.
- Closing your eyes serves a vital purpose; it blocks out all distractions the eyes always seem to want to look at. Plus, it forces you to focus more with your mind on what your breath is doing. Moreover, you can better keep your relaxation in check; tightness hinders breathing.
- Do not "hold your breath" at any point. There should be a natural, easy shift when transitioning between the inhale and exhale.
- Though you want to inhale as much as possible, do not do it to the point of straining when inhaling fully. Straining causes tightening, which may have a domino effect on surrounding muscles, ligaments, and veins. See the last sentence in the third indented paragraph above.

Now that all the checks and balances are covered, and you believe you are now ready, it is time to move on to the last instruction of this practice. I will give you fair warning, however, and it may be found in three related Scriptures, which I will give you momentarily. This is the warning: it may be better for you to repeat or stay a while longer in any of the prior steps than to venture into Step 5 at this time. It may be too challenging for you now, especially if you missed or lagged a little during the period of this entire sixty days of training. Get going with the next step only if you are firmly committed, can truly say, "I've got this!" and believe you need no further instruction in this unique breathing practice.

Once you move into the next step, or maybe I should say, once you are actively engaged in the next step, there are no additional instructions, and you will need to continue moving forward from all that you culled from steps 1 through 4 that highly improved your breathing, which helped you to be more calm and relaxed, and, with the forthcoming step 5, help put you in the zone where your emotions will no longer frazzle your nerves. Here is where you now need to focus on not turning back, three key words (terms):

1. No turning back (Luke 9:62).
2. Pick up step 5, and follow on (Luke 14:27).
3. Forget the past, and move ahead (Philippians 3:13).

Step 5:

Here is where you will put into effect all your steadfast training over the past two months that have brought you to this critical juncture. Here, you will not be diving off a springboard into a pool; you will be diving into the ocean of society, infested with everything mentioned in Romans 1:21–32 and what Paul calls a crooked and perverse generation, in Philippians 2:15. This time, however, you have available several contingencies that will both keep you afloat and protect you:

1. the perpetual correct breathing to calm and balance emotions
2. the word of God
3. the gift of faith God gave to you
4. DASA

A. Take ten to twenty seconds for one set (inhale/exhale), completing twenty sets after your daily morning communion with your Father. By the way, this communication is popularly known as prayer. Never, ever start a breathing session without giving Him first priority. Remember, it is His breath you breathe (Genesis 2:7). Also, compare Psalm 104:29.
B. Intermittently, throughout the day, seven days a week, practice several (five or more) sets of breathing in addition to the morning, noon, and night practice of twenty sets each.

DASA (DYNAMIC APPLICATION OF SPIRITUAL AWARENESS)

C. Perpetually engage in Step 5 until you go home to be with the Lord, or until 1 Thessalonians 4:15–18, whichever occurs first.

That concludes the instruction in breathing. As you continue, you will notice how your body defaults to inferior breathing. This is why it is vitally necessary to adhere to Step 5 until it becomes as automatic as inferior breathing. Over time, you will notice that the "lightheadedness" you felt when you first started practicing is actually the rejuvenation of brain cells. Additionally, you should notice less sleepiness at inappropriate times and consistently feel refreshed. Correct breathing will become so natural to you that you will find yourself doing it practically all day, every day, to the point where the morning, noon, and night practice will no longer be necessary. However, be advised, that it may take several years to reach that level. Remember, nothing good comes cheap and easy. Lastly, as you add this to the progress you have already made, do not think, *Oh, this is going to be so difficult.* That mindset is negative. Instead, think positively, as encouraged in Philippians 4:8.

May the Godhead strengthen you with His power so you will have the endurance and patience you need.

Chapter 4

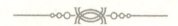

DASA at Work

In the last few chapters, you learned about the essence of DASA and how breathing is central to it, relative to its operation in association with the body. As a spiritual process activated only through the gift of faith that comes from God, DASA is detached from human emotion. To give you more clarity, DASA is an invisible quality empowered by the Holy Spirit who creates a holy temple within you to guide you toward holiness (1 Corinthians 6:19; Hebrews 12:14).

It is not instantaneous. Putting DASA-breathing into use is a gradual process that helps calm and relax your body, while at the same time, a calm, relaxed body allows DASA to excel and strengthen. This cannot be understood, however, with mere human (worldly) wisdom. Only when you allow yourself to be led by the Holy Spirit and begin living a God-centered lifestyle (Romans 8:5; Galatians 5:16) will you comprehend this profound truth.

DASA and the word of God are actually two sides of the same coin, both of which hinge on faith. Though I coined the acronym, DASA, in its essence, comes from the sword of the Spirit (Ephesians 6:17), and this *sword* can only be comprehended by applying it moment to moment (dynamically) by faith to your spiritual awareness. And so that you will not think all this is some form of mystical, mental gymnastics, or hocus-pocus, DASA manifests itself in physical action (Luke 11:28; James 1:22) (i.e., the spiritual awareness dynamically applied solely in your thoughts is nothing in and of

DASA (DYNAMIC APPLICATION OF SPIRITUAL AWARENESS)

itself). As the two Scriptures show, DASA must translate into what can actively be seen by others.

Another way to look at DASA is by noticing that the word of God is its *heart*. Your heart is alive and powerful; it pulls in old blood, nourishes it, and pumps out newly rejuvenated blood that travels throughout the entirety of the human body, working to spread this nourishment to benefit the body. The word of God is continual spiritual rejuvenation as you study the word, and as you gradually mature in it (Proverbs 2:1–2). You begin dynamically applying wisdom to your own life as you share your godly knowledge to benefit other saints and spread the gospel while engaging in godly work for the Lord.

Scriptures for DASA

The contents of this book will be useless to you if you do not make the effort to read each Scripture reference as you come to it. Over time, you will be able to appropriately apply Scriptures as necessitated by whatever difficulties you may encounter.

The word of God brings spiritual understanding and awareness. And God commands His saints to use that awareness by applying it to an ongoing lifestyle of good works in service to Him, who gives you eternal life, as shown in 2 Timothy 3:17. Scripture gives examples of the use and application of talents or experiences He blessed you with (Romans 12:6–8). And remember what Jesus, our Lord, said. He said, "The harvest is great, but the workers are few" (Matthew 9:37). So think of ways to motivate fellow saints to acts of love and good works (Hebrews 10:24). There are about eight billion people on planet Earth; only a fraction of them are true Christ-followers. If I could help one million souls become highly interested in DASA, and motivated to get seriously involved in engaging the practice of it, and each of them help motivate just two others, that would total three million souls for Christ. Sure, that's only a pittance in comparison to those billions of others. But it's enough to joyfully rock heaven according to Luke 15:7. So do it! Take to heart what I am sharing and *follow me* (John 13:17, 20)!

With the truth you receive from the word of God, you will also be exposed to the campaign messages of many politicians running for various offices who are not true believers or participants in God's word. In strategic efforts to capture your votes, they fill you full of idealistic rhetoric, painting a false vision in your mind, to the applause and cheers of those they dupe. Moreover, our institutions of higher learning are being taken over by liberal intellectuals who blot out any inkling of spiritual knowledge, exchanging it with philosophical conjecture, high-flown rhetoric, and vain human thinking spawned by the spiritual god of this world, rather than from Christ.

Even Christian educational institutions are being hijacked. Using an expression from Andrew Brunson,[3] they "compromise, dilute, and devalue" the educational integrity of students. Even worse is the forced inclusion of LGBTQ+-generated "educational material." And Dr. David Jeremiah shares, "We have deliberately turned away from God's original design for us."[4]

When I was young, a popular recording group, Earth, Wind & Fire, recorded a hit song entitled "That's The Way Of The World." According to the word of God, Satan, the devil, is the god of this world (2 Corinthians 4:4; Revelation 20:3).

Yet the world, in all its revelry, thinks they are having the time of their lives because two of the deceptive tactics the devil uses are as follows:

1. He dangles worldly treasures to attract you (Luke 4:5–7).
2. He impersonates light to hide his wicked, scheming darkness (2 Corinthians 11:14).

And when you look closely, you notice that billions of people love the way of the world with all their collective heart, soul, and strength. This is totally opposite of what Almighty God says

---

[3] Andrew Brunson, "Andrew Brunson: Be Faithful With No Regrets," *Decision Magazine*, (December 2022).

[4] Dr. David Jeremiah, *Angels: Who They Are and How They Help…What the Bible Reveals* (Multnomah 2006).

DASA (DYNAMIC APPLICATION OF SPIRITUAL AWARENESS)

(Deuteronomy 6:5). Jesus wholeheartedly supported this in Matthew 22:37.

God Himself is light; no darkness is in Him (1 John 1:5). And treasures are procured through Christ because they are guaranteed, safe, protected, and eternally preserved for us in the true place of our citizenship (Philippians 3:20). DASA is the means by which you know God's light is in you through Christ (John 3:21). And since you are made complete in Christ (Colossians 2:9–10), you are children of the light (John 12:36). This is the genuine light you use to counter the devil's artificial light. Anytime anyone comes at you with the darkness of false religion, humanistic ideology, LGBTQ agenda, or anything else contrary to the word of God, which is the Holy Spirit's sword, you need to unsheathe that glittering weapon, letting the brilliant light of truth beam all over that darkness (1 Timothy 6:16); make them flee from the holy light of God. Dr. David Jeremiah says, "[God is] sublimely and majestically holy—awesomely holy."[5] When all is said and done, there will be only one source of natural, divine light (Revelation 21:23).

DASA is the means by which you should be compelled to put the command of God (Matthew 22:37) into action. Loving Him with enthusiasm makes you treasure the word of truth that provides spiritual growth (Proverbs 2:1; 7:1–2). The truth of God's word flowing into you produces a heavenly vault of treasure for you (Matthew 6:19–21). Why would anyone even want the limited, contaminated worldly treasures over the pure, zero-defect, endless treasures Christ offers (Ephesians 3:8; Colossians 2:3)? Unfortunately, for those who do have wealth, it is not tenable, especially if you spend it on show-off worldly pleasures and vile, immoral activities (1 Timothy 6:17; James 5:1–3).

God's Payment

When a company pays a person a high starting bonus—recording artist, actor, sports figure, author, motivational speaker, etc.—

---

[5] Ibid.

you become indebted to that company to work for it and perform at your best in whatever the company expects of you. If you shirk your part of the deal or don't perform as expected, it is a breach of contract, and you are virtually robbing the company or cheating it out of its trusted investment in you.

In view of that, God paid a very high price for you; and this was an upfront payment for which He expected you to honor Him (1 Corinthians 6:20; 9:23), and not be tangled up and enslaved to the world. He actually purchased you to be His own people so that He could shower you with kindness, understanding, and wisdom, and give you the awesome privilege of being an heir to receive an inheritance of out-of-this-world riches (Ephesians 1:7, 14). God's payment freed us from slavery; we were slaves to Satan. As a matter of fact, it was a ransom God paid (Colossians 1:14; 1 Peter 1:18–19).

It is a sad state of affairs, though, when you see the lifestyle and notice the social integrity of the millions of people professing to be Christians. Not only are they robbing God as shown in Malachi 3:8–9, but they act practically like the unbelievers in the society (world) surrounding them. They invest exponentially more time, energy, and money into this pleasure-seeking world and its circumstances than in the kingdom of God. His word warns you over and over again to cease, halt, and stop participating "happy-go-lucky" throughout your life in this contumacious world-system. Dr. Luke, in Luke 12:31, tells you what to seek above all else.

This is what DASA *is all about: the breathing practice*; it prepares you bodily, while your spiritual awareness operates unhindered in that stress-free body. Remember, when you allow your negative emotions to control you, they wreak havoc mentally, psychologically, and physically, in addition to causing erratic breathing to your already oxygen-depleting *lazy breathing*. For enhanced benefits both physically and spiritually, you need to make DASA breathing a part of your daily lifestyle as you mature in Christ. Giving in to your emotions and lazy breathing depletes you of a significant amount of the oxygen the Godhead breathed into you in Genesis 2:7. You also short-circuit everything He is doing through you spiritually. So stay

DASA (DYNAMIC APPLICATION OF SPIRITUAL AWARENESS)

in the breath so you may always be mentally centered and spiritually focused on Christ.

Sanctified?

There is an ignorance about this word that precedes itself. So many believers blurt out, "I'm sanctified! Hallelujah!" Yet they have no idea what it means. I'm speaking of not a few, but millions of saints. I am not criticizing or faulting them; I'm simply making a statement of truth. Furthermore, an equal number of saints do not know where to look if they were asked, for example, to turn to the book of Ephesians. They page through the Old Testament attempting to find it. And I'm talking about those who have been saints for years. So please, do a fellow believer a favor; share this topic with him, her, or them.

Once someone listens to the word of God, and those *spiritual seeds* sprout in the heart, God gives the gift of faith to that person, and he or she, in turn, uses that faith to obey Romans 10:9–10. Seeing that their heart is true, God accepts them as His child (John 1:12), and they are considered "born again" (John 3:3). The Godhead (Father, Son, and Holy Spirit) "sanctifies" you at that point. What that clearly means is that He sets you aside from the unbelievers of the world to make you His holy temple. He can now live in you because you are now Holy Spirit–infused through Christ Jesus to the glory of the Father. To clarify that, God the Father enters you (1 Corinthians 3:16), the Holy Spirit enters you (1 Corinthians 6:19), and the Son enters you (2 Corinthians 13:5) (also see Galatians 4:6).

From those Scriptures, we may rightly conclude that the Godhead in all His fullness is in us, as corroborated by Colossians 2:9–10. When you study the word of God in this way, connecting them together and noticing how they harmoniously support one another with absolutely no contradiction, you are dynamically applying this truth to your spiritual awareness. In fact, so that you may be able to look at a group like 1 Corinthians 3:16 and 6:19 as well as Galatians 4:6, you might want to get a small notebook or use a computer or digital tablet, and title it Group Scriptures, or Harmonious

Scriptures, or whatever, and add some of these to it as well as others you discover yourself as you invest time studying and meditating on the word.

Holiness

Briefly, we covered *light, treasure,* and *payment or ransom.* You also now understand sanctification. And being in DASA mode means becoming familiar with the Scriptures, or some of them, that support you being holy. First of all, fully realize there is no type of clothing, no fasting, no pious-looking face, or no labor you can do to earn it—none!

Here is how it all comes about. Follow along very carefully, reading and pondering each Scripture reference. How about us calling this a *spiritual chain of events*? It all starts with somehow, somewhere, you read, hear, or see some Christian material—a book, magazine, Bible, radio, CD, Internet, TV, a Christian event, or perhaps a Christian crusade. The Father speaks to your heart through one or more of these sources, pointing you toward Jesus (John 6:44; 1 John 3:23). Then the Holy Spirit will *touch* your heart, like in Acts 2:36–41, for example. Nevertheless, upon creation, God created us as free moral agents. So individuals have the choice to accept or reject the Holy Spirit's prompting. Look at those who rejected Him (Acts 7:51–60).

So it was God who called you. In fact, believe it or not, He called you before you were born. Even more astonishing, He called you before even time began (1 Corinthians 1:2; Ephesians 1:4). The Father, awesome in holiness, is transcendent in holiness; even His name is holy (Leviticus 22:32; Psalm 99:3; Isaiah 6:3). No human being can endure the super intensity, glory, and light of His holiness (1 Timothy 6:16). And since God the Almighty Father Himself cannot die, He came down from heaven and veiled (hid) His intense brightness in a human body so we could look at Him, talk to Him, touch Him, experience His teaching and miracles. God named that human body Jesus (Luke 1:28–33), and it is the body He used to pay

DASA (DYNAMIC APPLICATION OF SPIRITUAL AWARENESS)

our ransom, reconcile sinful mankind to Himself, and make us holy (Colossians 1:22).

Stern Spiritual Warning

As you get started and begin growing in DASA, the first thing you need to prioritize at all times is that God called you to live a holy lifestyle, since He made you holy before the world was even created. If you willingly choose to turn back, then not only are you not fit for the kingdom of God, but you are also rejecting the Holy Spirit and are considered as a dog returning to its vomit (1 Thessalonians 4:7; 2 Peter 2:21–22). These dreadful Scriptures apply to a believer who disobeys God (2 Thessalonians 1:8–9; Hebrews 10:31; 12:29). So now after having received this living word of truth (Hebrews 4:12), there is no excuse for you to continue living in sin (John 15:22). Jesus gave up His divine rights (a form of self-denial) for you (Philippians 2:6–8), so you should reciprocate for Him (Luke 9:23; Romans 12:1). Now go forth in your DASA and be holy (1 Peter 1:15).

Chapter 5

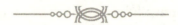

Connecting Scriptures

It took me several years of intensive study, praying for wisdom, and completing Bible study courses from three separate ministries before I felt completely relaxed and "at home" in the word of God, and communicating with my Father throughout the day and night, every single day. In fact, the Godhead set aside the last day (Saturday, a.k.a. the Sabbath) of the week as a holy day, not a *holiday*, to rest from normal occupations so that we may take time to worship Him as the living Father of all creation (Psalm 29:1–3; Hebrews 9:14). But by being in DASA mode 24-7, I have reached a point in my life where I do not typically dwell in a time mode or day-night-day mode as the average person does; to me, every single day, every hour, every moment is my *Sabbath* and in a constant state of being *in the moment* with Christ. I do not want to take up space here in this publication expounding on that. I may give more details in a future book.

Here in this chapter, rather than doing a discussion/Scripture reference, like I have done throughout this book, I have listed various Scriptures that dynamically support each other. To exercise and strengthen your DASA, you should read how the pairs or groupings are comparatively related to each other, meditate on them, write down any questions you come up with, and set them aside. In time, as you diligently study the word of God, you might be going over a Scripture(s), and the Holy Spirit may remind you of one of the questions you wrote down previously while providing the answer

DASA (DYNAMIC APPLICATION OF SPIRITUAL AWARENESS)

right there in what you were going over. Since the Holy Spirit works in various ways, you might hear the answer at a church sermon, a weekday Bible study, or in casual gospel conversation with a friend or friends.

One good thing about being in DASA mode is that I do not wait for a certain time of day or night to pray. I am spontaneous in my communication with my Father at any time, at any moment! Sometimes I simply sing a praise song, and that's it (Psalm 146:1–2; Psalm 147:1). DASA influences you powerfully as you become more aware that the Father and Jesus are in you (John 14:23, meaning the "Us" of Genesis 1:26 is living in you, which solidifies 1 John 4:4). When you realize who's got your back, there isn't any other person or force in the universe that should be able to "shake your tree."

The Holy Spirit just prompted me. Before I give you those paired and grouped Scriptures, it is to your advantage that I take one particular grouping and go over it with you. They involve the new life one has in Christ after that person accepts Him as his/her Savior and makes the Romans 10:9 confession of faith. Just like Jesus pointed out to a highly educated, influential religious leader who appeared befuddled about being born again, I must also clarify for you any misconceptions you may have, or any wrongly explained teaching you may have come across about this important subject. You will see for yourself relevant Scriptures strongly supporting this, which so many leaders misunderstand. After you see the validity of what I reveal to you, we may proceed to the listing of the paired and grouped Scriptures.

Let's go ahead and start at the source, which is John 3:3. Mostly everyone knows that Scripture, and the influential religious leader's human-minded response to a spiritual statement. It is what Jesus explains to Nicodemus after that (John 3:5–8), which had this respected-among-peers ruler scratching his head in verse 9. And Jesus chides him afterward. So it is actually verses 5 to 7 I am going to center on, which many fine Bible teachers seem to misunderstand. I have listened to some of them attempting to explain this spiritual concept with human reasoning. Then I will show you something profound about verse 11 that nearly everyone simply overlooks, especially if they have Bible versions that do not care enough to capitalize the first letter of pronouns relative to members of the Godhead.

To give you a much broader understanding of what I will show you in John 3:5–7, let's quickly skim some other relevant Scriptures. In Matthew 5:29–30, Jesus is not condoning self-mutilation, as it does nothing to change a person's heart. He uses such a graphic illustration to stress the seriousness of turning away from sin. In John 2:19–20, the so-called intelligent elite of the religious leaders showed their ignorance in their lack of comprehension. When Jesus used the word *this*, it was to direct attention to Himself, as verse 21 shows. Now on this next Scripture, there are large religious churches and groups today operating under the banner of Christianity that really teach their congregants they are actually eating the raw flesh of Jesus and drinking His blood (John 6:53–58). Satan has them deceived, and they cannot comprehend the implied spiritual significance, like the example in John 7:37–39.

And that brings us back to John 3:5, where Jesus speaks of water and the Spirit. Contrary to what others may teach, Jesus is using *water* as a metaphor for the word of God. John 15:3 says we are cleansed (purified, washed) by the word. John 17:17 and 19 says we are made holy by the word of truth. Apostle Paul speaks of Jesus's sacrifice to make the church holy and clean, washed by the cleansing of God's word (Ephesians 5:26). In a letter Paul wrote to one of his companions, he mentions new birth and life through the Holy Spirit (Titus 3:5). Another apostle also alludes to the word of God and water (1 Peter 1:23). There are many others you will see as you excel in DASA. One important thing to do is take notes when listening to preachers or Bible teachers so you may check up on their message in your own personal study time, like the Bereans did in Acts 17:11. All in all, when the word of God (water) and the Holy Spirit come together in your heart, the result is a spiritual birth.

Regarding the profoundness in John 3:11, here is what believers overlook—the word *We*. Again, if your Bible does not have the first letter of pronouns relating to Deity, or the Divine nature of Jesus capitalized, then it is easy to become confused as to who's who. Perhaps you should have an NKJV translation available in addition

DASA (DYNAMIC APPLICATION OF SPIRITUAL AWARENESS)

to whatever translation you favor. So now that I have pointed it out to you, who do you think Jesus is referring to? He can't be talking about His disciples, because up to then, they were new apprentices. Jesus also mentions the word *Our*. He could not have been talking about angels; they were not walking around giving testimonies. How about any of the prophets of old? Not them either; they all died centuries prior to Jesus's lifetime on earth.

Come now with me to Psalm 2:2–3. In verse 3, it speaks of *Their* chains. I will help you out not by simply giving you an overt answer. But what I will do is answer indirectly to give you the chance to use DASA to determine the answer. I am going to pearl-string some Scriptures as your indirect answer:

- Genesis 3:22, 11:7
- Isaiah 6:8
- John 14:23
- 2 Corinthians 13:14
- Colossians 2:9

There are indeed many, many more, but these should provide some beneficial perusal and contemplation for you. Enjoy!

Scripture Pairs and Groups

A fruit that the Godhead created, sized to be held in your hand, has a softish interior, comes in green, yellow, or even a reddish-yellow color, is very nutritious, and is deliciously sweet, is the pear. You like them, right? Well, you are in for a delicious, spiritually nutritious treat. But you need to trust God and His word rather than your human understanding, then you will have healing and bodily strength (Psalm 119:103; Proverbs 3:5, 8). So go ahead and *pluck 'n' eat* these spiritual *pears*.

- First of all, relax and be at peace (John 14:27; Philippians 4:7).
- Be full of joy in Christ (John 15:11; 1 Peter 1:8).

37

- The New Testament was concealed in the Old Testament, and then the Old Testament was revealed in the New Testament. One of the mysteries is Christ lives in you (Ephesians 3:17; Colossians 1:27).
- Almighty God told the people of Israel through Moses that He is "I AM." Myriad centuries later, Jesus told the powerful religious leaders of His era that He Himself was "I AM" (Exodus 3:14; John 8:58). So who's who?
- Moses, who was a prophet, speaks of the Lord as the Father in Deuteronomy 32:6. A different prophet over seven hundred years later called a yet-to-be-born Baby, which he never saw, "everlasting Father" (Isaiah 9:6).
- According to John 6:63, only the Holy Spirit gives eternal life. But the Lord (Jesus) says He gives eternal life in John 10:28. So are there two Beings doling out eternal life, both Jesus and the Holy Spirit? Here is a hint (2 Corinthians 3:17).
- Jesus, in His resurrected body, spoke from heaven to Paul. He spoke as "I AM" to Moses (Exodus 3:14; John 8:58). When Jesus appeared to Moses, it was evincive of an Angel in flaming fire (Exodus 3:2). However, it was intensely blinding light to the apostle Paul (Acts 9:3; 1 Timothy 6:16). I gave you that for explanation. Now here's the juicy pairs you may bite (Exodus 3:2–6 and Acts 9:3–5).
- Evinced as a "rock," Jesus followed the Israelites in the wilderness. Moreover, He lived within the Old Testament prophets. Don't take my word for it, though. Let these golden pairs enlighten you (1 Corinthians 10:4; 1 Peter 1:11).
- Are you aware that Christ-followers are not of this world? Taste these two very sweet pairs (John 15:19 and Philippians 3:20).
- First place is *first place*, period! No one is before; no one's beside. If someone was beside you, wouldn't that qualify as a tie? And whoever is last is last; no one's after that. Well, Almighty God Himself claimed both first and last, as well

DASA (DYNAMIC APPLICATION OF SPIRITUAL AWARENESS)

as saying there's no other God. Guess what? Someone challenges that bold averment. Could there be a possible heavenly tie? See for yourself (Isaiah 44:6 and Revelation 1:17).

- Incongruent to the church Jesus founded (Matthew 16:18), numerous religions abound. Not quite a few of them speak of the Holy Spirit as simply a wind, or some type of energetic force. Acts 5:3 and 13:2 are two succulent pairs proving them wrong—and here's a bonus (Romans 8:26).

- Now take a spiritual bite of these related pairs (Exodus 20:1–17; Galatians 3:24–25). Through Moses, God made the Ten Commandments an explicit mandate which extended to Christ's crucifixion. It was the written letter of the law, whereas disobedience meant subsequent death (Hebrews 10:28). Contrarily, through the death of Jesus, the written letter of the law was implicitly subsumed by the new covenant of grace, leading us to Romans 3:8 and 10. And as having become born anew in Christ (2 Corinthians 5:17), the Lord ascribes His laws in our minds and writes them on our hearts (Hebrews 8:10). May Christ, who dwells within you (2 Corinthians 13:5), enlighten you to this profound truth.

That should be enough *pairs* to pique your interest and give you the desire to discover more for yourself in God's awesome word of truth. There simply is no other book on planet Earth as powerfully and spiritually profound that can match the unmatched word of God (i.e., the Holy Bible).

My deep desire is that this publication serves as a tool to motivate my fellow saints to faithful good works in Christ (Hebrews 10:24). May anyone who has never chosen to follow Jesus make your confession as the Scriptures show in Romans 10:9–10. Now not later is *the best* time to begin a new life living in the Spirit of God (Galatians 5:16, 25). To show you how much God truly loves you and wants to forgive you, do yourself a favor and read Psalm 103:12 and Isaiah 1:18–20, 43:25, and 55:6–7. After letting that sink in, go and read John 3:16 and 17:20–23.

Groupies

Nearly all "hot" singers, bands, or movie stars have their share of fans or groupies. Well, here's a secret I want to share with you. Many groupies abound in the most popular book on Earth, authored by a consortium of people, from highly educated to those with negligible education, from wealthy, powerful kings to poor shepherds and fishermen, even a physician is included as a major contributing co-author, all of whom were inspired, empowered, and overseen by the Godhead (Matthew 22:43–44; 2 Timothy 3:16–17; 2 Peter 1:20–21). Being translated into thousands of the world's languages and dialects shows the sheer popularity of the word of God. With that said, I hope these Scripture groupies contribute to your dynamic application of spiritual awareness (DASA).

Help those who are downright poor, or experiencing difficulty (Psalm 41:1; Proverbs 11:24; 14:21; 17:2; 19:17; 21:13; 22:9; 28:27; 1 John 3:17).

The Godhead, who is omnipotent and omniscient, knows your thoughts (Psalm 7:9; Jeremiah 11:20; 17:10; Ezekiel 11:5; Luke 16:15; Romans 2:16; Hebrews 4:12; Revelation 2:23).

God does not shift like a shadow, changing His mind like mere humans, and it is impossible for Him to lie. That is why Proverbs 3:5 was written, and why Jesus made His statements in Matthew 4:4 and John 6:27. Here are the groupies (Numbers 23:19; 1 Samuel 15:29; Psalm 89:34–35; Psalm 93:5; Isaiah 40:9; Ezekiel 24:14; Malachi 3:6; Titus 1:2; Hebrews 6:17–18; James 1:17).

Immerse yourself in those groups often, spending significant time allowing them to become rooted in your mind. Don't look at investing time in reading and studying God's word as though it is a not-too-well-liked chore. Learn to desire it with eagerness and excitement. I even composed a song about it; it's an upbeat one entitled, "Cruise in the Word of God." Maybe you will hear it sooner or later.

When you allow the word of God to strengthen your DASA, you begin to be transformed by the power of the Godhead working within you, helping you to truly understand His word, His will, and His purpose for your life, which They had already predetermined

DASA (DYNAMIC APPLICATION OF SPIRITUAL AWARENESS)

even before saying "Let Us" as shown in Genesis 1:26. The word of God, the Father, and the Holy Spirit, all point you to Jesus (Luke 24:44; John 16:13–14; 1 John 3:23). And Jesus is the embodiment of the Godhead (Colossians 2:9), so when you "put off" your sinful lifestyle (James 1:21) and "put on" Christ as expressed in Romans 13:14 and Galatians 3:27, you are strapped—suited and booted!

Now through these groupies, you will learn much about the holy fire of the Godhead; it can bring salvation, it can heal, or it can destroy and kill (Genesis 3:24; Exodus 3:2; 13:21; 19:18; 2 Kings 2:11; 6:17; Isaiah 66:15–16; Matthew 3:11; 2 Thessalonians 1:8; 2 Peter 3:10; Revelation 20:14; 21:8).

Of the various qualities pointed out by Jesus for saints to project, forgiveness is one that is paramount. So much emphasis is placed on it that it is magnified in the epistles of the apostles, with John giving forgiveness special attention.

I tell you this with all the seriousness I can muster; if you will not forgive everyone who has ever said bad things about, cursed you, and done any wrong to you or your loved ones, then your guaranteed destiny is Revelation 19:12 and 14 because of the Lord's statement of truth in Matthew 6:15. So before you decide to risk not forgiving anyone, consider the ridicule, scorn, hatred, hostility, beatings, sheer torture, and crucifixion Jesus endured. Yet He showed supreme love as He hung on rough, splintered wood, His tortured body all black and blue, swollen, bloodied, and through gargling blood probably in His throat, He still said from His dying heart, "Father, forgive them because they don't know what they're doing."

So here! Take these groups and refer to them often in DASA. And remember God's forgiveness to you is a love gift (2 Chronicles 7:14; Psalm 103:3, 12; Isaiah 43:25; Jeremiah 31:34; Matthew 6:14–15; Mark 11:25; Luke 23:34; Romans 5:15; Colossians 2:13; 3:13; 1 John 2:2).

One of the most difficult things for believers to latch onto, and that hinders them, is faith and doubt. They do not cling to that precious gift God freely gives us because they let doubt come and snatch it away. Just think, people put practically 100 percent trust in worldliness and human promises, but when Jesus says to ask (pray for something) in faith, and believe in your heart it will happen, with no doubts whatsoever, you seem to have a problem with that. Or when He tells you to deny yourself and put Him first (Luke 9:23), you balk. That is why the New Testament is replete with numerous situations regarding faith.

Be mindful of these three important things:

1. You become righteous with God through faith (Romans 3:30).
2. You receive the Holy Spirit through faith (Galatians 3:14).
3. It is absolutely impossible to please God without faith (Hebrews 11:6).

DASA is foundational in putting your faith into practice. Besides those three, I will just give you these few groups, and refer you to Romans and Hebrews to receive a smorgasbord of faith (Ephesians 4:5; 6:16; 1 John 5:4).

When the devil tempted Jesus in the desert wilderness after He was famished, besides being hot, stinking, sweaty, and dirty, Jesus didn't check the government-mandated laws and say, "Oh, the Old Testament laws are outdated, so I can't use them." Instead, He took what was written many centuries prior and flung it at Satan (e.g., Matthew 4:10; Deuteronomy 6:13). If millions of today's saints could be in DASA mode, together we could do the same when society tries to tell us the word of God is outdated, and that we need to accept all the laws enacted giving LGBTQ proponents more freedom to perpetuate their flagrant immorality upon the whole of society.

It appears that the ungodly activities of the LGBTQ society are attempting to turn the world into one global Sodom and Gomorrah. Numerous people worldwide are joining their ranks, with untold thousands allowing themselves to be what they call "transgendered," as well as lobbying politicians to pass laws forcing medical institutions to participate in their perversion by providing what they neologize to be gender-affirming care. With the passage of such laws, the leaders try to make us believe they are promoting equality. In

DASA (DYNAMIC APPLICATION OF SPIRITUAL AWARENESS)

reality, however, their self-centered laws are a total contradiction to Almighty God's laws.

Because of a contumacious mindset and bias against biblical morality, there are rapes, fornication, adultery, widespread pornography, mass shootings, social disunity, political corruption, AIDS, Ebola, COVID-19, monkeypox, famine, and all of the societal ills shown in Romans 1:28–32, 1 Corinthians 6:9–10, Galatians 5:19–21, Ephesians 5:5, 2 Thessalonians 1:8, 1 Timothy 1:10, and 2 Timothy 3:1–5. Of these groups of Scriptures, everything listed is happening to such a degree that it is unprecedented since the creation of the world. And the only thing all the most sophisticated technology of so-called high-IQ people and scientists have done is to make sin even more prevalent. Regarding all of this, John 7:7 informs us of why Jesus Christ is so hated.

Initially, the devil started out perfect and holy when the Godhead created him, giving him the angelic name of Lucifer. He was created as one of the highest-ranking angels with exceptional beauty, talent, along with free will. Unfortunately, he allowed his beauty and talent to go to his head, which led to selfish pride and arrogance. With his "me, me, me" attitude, he was not content with what God created him to be. So he overstepped his boundary, became bold, and recruited a third of heaven's angels to join him in taking over. And that sort of insolent pride is what brought about his downfall along with his angelic cronies (Isaiah 14:12; Ezekiel 28:11–19; Luke 10:18; 2 Peter 2:4; Jude 6; Revelation 12:3).

The mindset and actions of the LGBTQ+ community follows the pattern of their father the devil who recruited a specific number of angels to support his devious treason and attempted coup d'é tat (John 8:44; Revelation 12:7–9). Here on earth, the devil supernaturally works in the minds and hearts of those who reflect the gospel of Christ; he blinds their spiritual eyes to the truth as he recruits them from every nation under the sun (2 Corinthians 4:4; Ephesians 2:2; 6:12; 1 Peter 5:8).

The reality is that the LGBTQ+ community replaces God and His holy standards of righteous behavior (Ephesians 1:4; 1 Thessalonians 4:7–8) with their pursuit of perverted sexual immorality and gender-changing, hoping a life of satisfaction may be found in that. It is a complete rejection of Almighty God. In essence, their waywardness is tantamount to them delving into witchcraft and idol worship. According to the gospel of God (Romans 1:1), which reflects the gospel of Christ (Romans 1:16), rebellion against Him is witchcraft, and stubbornness is viewed as idol worship (1 Samuel 15:23; Colossians 3:5–6).

I hope you can see the urgency of practicing and growing in the dynamic application of spiritual awareness so that you will not be ensnared by worldly idolatry and witchcraft of a contumacious society (Romans 12:2; 1 Corinthians 7:23; James 4:4; 1 John 2:15–17).

Two things separate people from the holiness of the Almighty Creator: (1) evil thoughts; (2) evil actions. The two may potentially become one according to Matthew 5:28 and James 1:14–15. As you grow in your DASA, exceeding importance is placed on holiness. Why? Because Scripture says that without it, you will never enter into God's presence (Hebrews 12:14). In being holy, you let your lifestyle be governed by the gospel of the Lord Jesus (Ephesians 5:15), and not by the shifting laws of a degenerate society, you show a distinction between them and you as a child of a holy, Almighty God.

God Himself wrapped a body of human flesh (Jesus) around His own Spirit so that He could use it as a onetime sacrifice for our sins and make us righteous by virtue of His holiness to present us to Himself as faultless (Ephesians 1:4–5; Colossians 1:22). Do you see and understand the profoundness of God's unselfish act? Do you comprehend the Godhead? As you know, the Godhead is the Father, the Holy Spirit, and Christ—one God! And we come to the Father, through the Holy Spirit, because of Christ (John 14:6; Ephesians 2:18; Hebrews 7:25). That is why we are complete when we stay rooted in Christ (Colossians 2:9). And that is why you need DASA to keep you aware that you are a foreigner here on earth (Hebrews 13:14). When we arrive *home*, we will never again remember this life on earth (Isaiah 65:17).

DASA (DYNAMIC APPLICATION OF SPIRITUAL AWARENESS)

The Throne

The Scriptures give us many vivid details about the throne of our Creator. As for me, all the suffering, the tribulations and trials, and the hardships I go through here on earth pale in comparison to the sounds, sights, and treats waiting for me near God's throne. Enduring the difficulties here is worth the *price* of admission there. But I greatly praise and thank the Lord that He has already paid it forward. That includes a spectacular, "out-of-this-world" place He prepared for me (John 14:1–3). Imagine that! God Himself is going to show me around my brand *spanking* new place (Revelation 21:3, 5).

Best of all, I won't have to worry about a utility bill anymore; my Father's own glory is going to light that place up. I'm urbanized, so city life is what I enjoy. No need for me to even think about going to the jewelry store. My place will be surrounded by every type of precious jewel one can imagine; and get a load of this—even the main street is super pure gold, unlike anything here on earth. I'll be sitting comfortably in my place with a riverside view of the two trees of life on each side of the sparkling *water of life* river that flows from God's throne. I'll also love the trees because they will be producing twelve different types of fruit after each crop. And I'll be able to have a face-to-face dialogue with His Majesty there before His glorious throne.

Now take a look at some of the various descriptions about His throne: 2 Chronicles 18:18; Psalms 45:6, 47:8, 99:1, 102:12, and 103:19; Isaiah 6:1; 66:1; Daniel 7:9; Revelation 4:2–3; 20:11; 22:3. As you should have noticed, the Almighty has lots of various thrones.

There are quite a number of Scriptures about my Dad's own throne, but look at Psalm 103:19 and Isaiah 66:1. What! Yes, the entirety of heaven is His throne. Whatever the case may be, I stay in DASA mode every second of every day, 24-7. Someone might say, "But you don't have any time to *enjoy* life." What! Enjoy? You call this mess of society and this worldliness *life*? Well, I will say this to that. You go right ahead and disregard the Godhead's predestined purpose for your life as you *enjoy* cruising around in the quagmire of selfishness and splashing around in the pool of worldliness. As you are doing that, I will be cruising in the word of God and looking forward to splashing my feet in the Water of Life River and eating fruit unimaginably succulent and deliciously juicy. Too bad you will not be able to join me; Matthew 7:21–23 lets you know why.

Actually, all I am explaining to you is infinitesimally minute and impossible to accurately convey in any human language because unbelievers are unable to comprehend the magnitude of what Christ-followers, in the strength of DASA, can spiritually discern. So for the sake of believers, I will continue on.

Sitting by the river of life, chilling out might be cool, but I would rather be where the real action is happening. As a matter of fact, I am going to work as hard as I can for the Lord here on earth so I may be eligible for some of the rewards He will be doling out to hard workers who stay the course, remaining faithful and victorious (Revelation 3:20–21; 22:12). I won't even bother commenting on those two Scriptures because they mean exactly what they say.

Crowns and Rewards

Since I am not a thief, I won't steal away the excitement you will get by studying the word of God yourself to learn all you can about crowns. I will share some groups on rewards, as they are relevant to this current discussion (Isaiah 49:4; Matthew 5:12; Luke 6:35; Ephesians 6:8).

According to the prophet Isaiah and the last New Testament apostle, John, all the action is happening around His Holiness seated on His majestic throne. Isaiah and John explain the same sight in two different ways. Isaiah talks briefly about seeing the Lord sitting on a throne, while six-winged seraphim catered to Him. John gives a rather detailed explanation of that throne when he says, "One sat on the throne," and John speaks of six-winged "living beings." Both Isaiah and John say the same thing regarding what they heard, however; the seraphim, or living beings, were exclaiming: "Holy, holy, holy," giving reverent praise to the Lord God Almighty.

That is where the real action is going to be, and I hope one of my rewards will be a front-row seat near that throne. As Proverbs 3:5

DASA (DYNAMIC APPLICATION OF SPIRITUAL AWARENESS)

commands, I put all my trust in the Godhead, and I will continue in DASA mode while letting it reflect in all my physical actions so that when the Lord judges my work, I will be rewarded accordingly (2 Corinthians 5:10; Revelation 20:12).

It boggles my imagination to think about the incredible, holy-awesome action that will take place around the throne on that great coronation day of Jesus (Philippians 2:10–11). That's why I am not afraid or ashamed to do what Colossians 3:1–2 says. Another Scripture you may want to add to this reward-grouping is Hebrews 13:14. I am also overjoyed at how I am going to arrive there, which is why, being in DASA mode, I have no fear of dying whatsoever. If I die before a certain, forthcoming event, no problem because an angel will immediately zip from heaven as I take my last breath. Then he, or they, will escort my spirit to heaven because I wouldn't know the way there through billions of miles of stars in the universe. However, if I'm living when that certain, forthcoming event happens, that's fine too. Either way, I have the assurance from the word of God, so I'll encourage you with this Scripture (1 Thessalonians 4:15–18). That is the event I was referring to.

Getting back to the throne action, the Apostle Paul was given a view of it as well. He was so mesmerized by the awesome glory there that he was at a loss for words to describe it (2 Corinthians 12:2–4). Isaiah gives you a taste in a few words (Isaiah 6:1–3). But the Apostle John makes me want to be seated at a front-row table because his explanation is served up like an elaborate, exquisite, white-glove, four-course meal, in Revelation chapters four and five; take a look for yourself. And with your help, together we may potentially motivate three million or more people to engage in DASA so they too can listen to the "new song" the heavenly hosts will sing (Revelation 5:9). Be blessed as you share connecting Scriptures with others.

Chapter 6

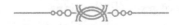

Abandoned

All of the postmodern world's increased human knowledge and incredible technological advances, although impressive and commendable, have never been able to change the heart of mankind, nor can they tame the human tongue (Matthew 15:19; James 3:5–10). Moreover, for thousands of years since mankind's existence, it is a proven fact that the behavior and customs of the world will never result in sustainable peace—ever! This is why the Godhead made the sword of the Spirit (Ephesians 6:17) so inclusive so that it could expose the condition of man's heart, and let them know of their need for a Savior. It also gives a fair warning for Christ-followers to refuse participation in worldliness (Acts 17:30; Romans 12:2; Galatians 1:4; Ephesians 4:23; 5:6–7).

No matter how much more sophisticated human technology becomes, the only thing man will ever succeed at is human speculation. They are woefully unable to disprove the Creator as an objective reality, so they dismiss Him as a matter of subjective preference. It is the sinful condition of their collective heart that keeps them glued to this unholy mindset, which makes it impossible to approach God's holiness. Sadly, all their faith, hope, and trust are focused on the limitation of what their finite minds can invent rather than trust in the holy God of all creation.

Holiness is an allusion to God's divine, unchangeable character. He is holy by virtue of His nature. Non-Christian religions of the

DASA (DYNAMIC APPLICATION OF SPIRITUAL AWARENESS)

world may consider their writings or religious artifacts and actions to be "holy," but this word came from the Almighty and is exclusive to Him only, as shown on the seventh day after creation (Genesis 2:3).

When the Godhead completed creating the universe, with Earth being the last planet, He was completely satisfied as He looked over the Earth and the male and female beings He *pulled* from the ground; the Father designed, the Word created, and the Holy Spirit empowered, and now sustains creation. Afterward, He mentally commented on how pleased He was with His creation (Genesis 1:31). The one Godhead, who perpetually operates in tripartite harmony, credits the Word with creating everything for His own purpose and holding it all together by His word (John 1:1–4; Colossians 1:15–17; Hebrews 1:3, 10). So the Word does it with His word. And the Word (who became Jesus) created everything for His own purpose or pleasure. Here are two Scriptures substantiating it (Psalm 33:6 and Romans 9:11, 17).

Every single thing, whether visible to the eyes or invisible (e.g., air), has a specific purpose for which the Godhead predetermined. And nothing in all the Godhead's creation has ever changed or "decided" to change from what He created it to be—except for humans. They chose instead to listen to their spiritual father, the devil, who dazzles them with "that's the way of the world" (Luke 4:5–7). With their tongues dangling like dogs, worldly people lap it up salaciously as they follow and worship Satan, while lavishly and ceaselessly investing in his kingdom. Because of the intense craving of people's self-centered hearts for the pleasures of this world, the Godhead had no choice but to hand them over (abandon them) to their ungodly desires and greed, as truthfully conveyed in Romans 1:24–28 (NLT).

> So God abandoned them to do whatever things their shameful hearts desired. As a result, they did vile and degrading things with each other's bodies. They traded the truth about God for a lie. So they worshiped and served the things God created instead of the Creator [Himself], who is

worthy of eternal praise! Amen. That is why God abandoned them to their shameful desires. Even the women turned against the natural way to have sex and instead indulged in sex with each other. And the men, instead of having normal sexual relations with women, burned with lust for each other. Men did shameful things with other men, and as a result of this sin, they suffered within themselves the penalty they deserved. Since they thought it foolish to acknowledge God, [He] abandoned them to their foolish thinking and let them do things that should never be done.

The current way of the world—unfriendliness, slander, betrayal, useless gossip, pride, lack of self-control, foolishness, young lust, fornication (sex-dating), adultery, transgendering, boasting, cruelty, disrespect to the elderly, being womanizers, recklessness, piousness, artificial Christianity, and every other worldly behavior contrary to the gospel of Christ—cannot coexist with the holiness of the Godhead. He must view us through Jesus to withstand the awesome glory of His holiness and stand in His presence (1 Timothy 6:16). Being "covered" in Christ does not make a person *good* per se (Psalm 14:2–3), but Christ is the Godhead's contingency plan, which He established even before the beginning of time (2 Corinthians 5:21; 2 Timothy 1:9).

The Lord's *reservation* has already been made for you; it is the *reservation of life*. But though it is there, it remains unreserved until you activate (accept) it by your faith, and it must be a moment-to-moment faith from the point you activate it until you take your last breath on this earth. This is what the Apostle Paul meant when he mentioned "faith to faith" in Romans 1:17. A minor Old Testament prophet says, "it is through faith that a righteous person has life" (Habakkuk 2:4 NLT).

Do not neglect the Godhead's divine contingency plan. Activate your reservation ASAP! Then begin engaging in DASA, which will help guide you in a godly lifestyle evidenced by good works. These

DASA (DYNAMIC APPLICATION OF SPIRITUAL AWARENESS)

good works will flow from your talent, experience, wealth, and resources, preparing you for an eternity with Jesus (Matthew 6:19–21; John 17:24). Dynamic application of spiritual awareness (DASA) is imperative in this time of spiritual decadence and social breakdown, whereby saints must strive to live by God's holy standards.

Because the Lord is both merciful and just, He is ever ready to forgive anyone of sin if they repent (have a true change of heart) and choose Jesus Christ (Psalm 86:5; Ephesians 1:7); the one and only "deadly" sin one absolutely will not be forgiven is shown in Matthew 12:31–32. And in all fairness, keeping things divinely equal, He must be just and not allow sin to perpetually flourish; eternal doom is the payday for all who choose to remain unrepentant and refuse to accept His offer of mercy, grace, and forgiveness through Christ Jesus (Psalm 62:12; Romans 2:5–11; 4:5). This *sweet-deal* offer is available to anyone and everyone reading this book who has not yet made the personal decision to choose the Lord Jesus Christ to save your soul from the dreaded White Throne Doomsday Judgment (Revelation 20:11–15). The holy word of God is final and unmovable (Matthew 24:35), so practice DASA as His word grows in your heart (Psalm 119:11). And in God's time, Revelation 21:3–7 will be your reward, and He will never abandon you.

Chapter 7

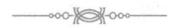

The Hated Jew

"I'm going full DEFCON 3 on Jewish people" appeared on a major social media platform in mid-2022 by a popular celebrity, causing a ruckus, heated debates, verbal attacks, finger-pointing, racial stereotyping, distorted truths, and severed business partnerships. Far from being new, this particular antisemitic threat, however, raised eyebrows and was a cause for concern because the hate-monger who posted it had a following, or viewership, of multiple millions. Ironically, the popular celebrity, a Black man, disregards being labeled antisemitic because "Black people are Jewish too." If that's the case, then Black people need to beware of him and proceed with caution, since his rant includes "Black people also who are Jews."

Here's the "kicker" regarding that post which inflamed many people. He who posted it claims to be a "born again Christian." Hmmm! We'll come back to that momentarily. Let's first put that social media, widely viewed, posting in check with a widely viewed *posting* by a popular Jewish man.

> In the same way, the tongue is a small thing that makes grand speeches. But a tiny spark can set a great forest on fire. And the tongue is a flame of fire. It is a whole world of wickedness, corrupting your entire body. It can set your whole life on

DASA (DYNAMIC APPLICATION OF SPIRITUAL AWARENESS)

fire, for it is set on fire by hell itself. (James 3:5–6 NLT)

When a baby is physically born, it becomes a family member. When one is spiritually born (born again), he or she becomes a family member (child of God). As a child of God, one must both speak and act with godly integrity, as well as "love each other with genuineness," as stated by another Jewish man in Galatians 5:14. From God Almighty's own mouth, a command was issued: "Love your neighbor as you love yourself. I am the Lord" (Leviticus 19:18). Keeping in mind the social media hate posting, "I'm going full DEFCON 3 on Jewish people," and his claim to be a "born again Christian," let's examine those two contrasting statements, against postings by two other Jews:

- Most important of all, continue to show deep love for each other, for love covers a multitude of sins (1 Peter 4:8).
- If someone says, "I'm a born again Christian," but hates others, that person is a liar; for if we don't love people we can see, how can we love God, whom we cannot see? (1 John 4:20)

Now the poster of that hateful social media content might be right about being born again, but it is born again to the synagogue of Satan (Revelation 2:9), not as a born again Christian; the Scriptures call him a liar.

Back in the 1950s and 1960s, Black people were negatively portrayed by the epithet "colored people." In this modern age, thinking they are using a new term, they want to be called "people of color." Duh! Colored people/people of color! Really? What color is sugar? What color is salt? What color is cotton in the pod? Doesn't that tell you something? So "people of color" undoubtedly includes White; white is a color. But whoever you are, whatever religious title you slap onto yourself, or whatever your "color," it has nothing to do with the condition of one's heart.

There are Black folks cheating, robbing, hurting, and killing other Blacks; there are Chinese destroying other Chinese; Filipinos fighting against their own countrymen; Islamic factions battle each other, e.g., Iran against Saudi Arabia. Whites contend with other Whites; Judaism Jews struggle with Christian Jews; Africans in Ethiopia, Sudan, and Johannesburg are slaughtering one another. That does not seem to register with people. Yet when someone of another color or race assaults one differently "colored," it all of a sudden changes to a racial aspect, with individuals stigmatizing an entire race of people for the actions of one or a few.

All of the above proves that the Scriptures are 100 percent accurate about the heart of humanity when they leave God out of their lives, neglect God's commands, disobey Him, or say they are believers of God or born again believers (Christians), but their lives (lifestyle) totally betray what they say with their lips (Genesis 6:5; Psalm 2:1–3; 36:1; Isaiah 29:13; Romans 1:29–31). Moreover, anyone who finds fault with the Jews, you'd better not tread water in that area, and you should guard your mouth very carefully before saying anything negative or hateful against them (Genesis 12:3; Matthew 7:1–5; Romans 2:1–3; James 4:11–12). Now if you are a Black person, and you have any dislike, discord, animosity, or hatred against Jews, then according to what that loser stated about "Black people are Jewish too," you hate yourself and other Black people.

Lastly, all of you who say you are Christian, born again believer, Christ-follower, or any other title related to Christ, if you do not have a heart for Jews, are indifferent toward them, do not support them with your prayers, time, or offerings, and/or you harbor within you any ill will, or you just don't care about them, then you may as well stop calling yourself a Christian, stop reading your Bible, do not pray to God anymore, and cease going to church. The reason why is because you are simply wasting your time. In fact, you are just boring God (Isaiah 1:12–15; 59:2–4). It is the condition of your heart, which contains resentment and discrimination toward Jews, that separates you from God, who does not look at the color of one's skin or their race (1 Samuel 16:7; Isaiah 11:3; Romans 2:11).

DASA (DYNAMIC APPLICATION OF SPIRITUAL AWARENESS)

The Jews (nation of Israel) are a nation of people God Almighty personally chose, beginning with one solitary man who was Abram (Genesis 12:1–3). It could have been any other person; African, Caucasian, Chinese, Arabian, Spanish, or anyone; He chose a Semitic person, however, because that's what He willed to do, and who are you to argue (Isaiah 45:9–11)?

- The Bible you read was written by (through) Jews.
- God clothed Himself in a Jewish body (John 1:14).
- He conducted His entire ministry in the Jewish nation of Israel.
- His earthly name was Jewish (Yeshua).
- The One who you depend upon for your eternal salvation is a Jew.
- And when He returns to set up His earthly kingdom, it will be headquartered in Jerusalem.

So as I said, you'd better think twice before harboring ill-conceived thoughts about God's hand-picked people because you are cursed by God Himself for doing so, and you would be foolish to be cursed by God (2 Thessalonians 1:8–9; Hebrews 10:31; 12:29). If you have read this and know in your heart you have treated Jews with contempt or discriminated against any other race of people different from yours, the Lord is merciful, just, and willing to forgive you, but only if your heart is truly repentant (Psalm 19:12; Isaiah 55:7; 66:2).

Now for those of you who are Jews by birth and have harbored bad feelings in your heart toward non-Jews because you believe God chose you only, and not Gentiles (non-Jews), you need to "wake up," repent (Psalm 51:17), and meditate on Romans 2:28–29. And going beyond that, under Christ, there is no Jew, there is no Gentile; there is just one family, which is the church (the body of Christ), and the more people that latch onto this truth, the less hatred there will be (Ephesians 2:14–22). Concentrate fastidiously on that Scripture; learn it forward, backward, and inside out until you are convinced in your heart that among all who have genuinely put their trust completely in Christ, there are no separate religions (Judaism/ Christianity) or denominations in Christ.

> For there is one body and Spirit… There is
> one Lord, one faith, one baptism, and one God
> and Father. (Ephesians 4:4–6)

More than anything else in life, the one you need to maintain a close, personal relationship with and commit your life to is the hated Jew: the Jew that Muslims don't accept; the Jew that Buddhists don't really know; the Jew that Communists ignore; the Jew that Jehovah's Witnesses say was a "created angel"; the Jew that atheists don't believe in; and the Jew that the world and Satan hate (John 7:7; 15:18), and it spills over onto us (1 John 3:13).

All true, committed Christ-followers will experience different types and levels of world hostilities, but learn the dynamic application of spiritual awareness fervently so it will help you to endure (Mark 13:13). And we Christ-followers should also pray for the peace of Jerusalem (Psalm 122:6–9).

Chapter 8

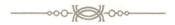

The Godhead

From eternity past, there has been the holy, harmonious unity of threeness in the Godhead. You will need to really lean on your dynamic application of spiritual awareness (DASA) to comprehend some profound highlights I share here. I say *highlights* because what is covered here only skims the surface, whereas the book I mentioned earlier will cover everything in explicit, detailed, never-before-seen profoundness.

As you may want to know, time, or what we know about time, did not begin until the rotation of the Earth (Genesis 1:5, 8, 13) after the Godhead created it. God gave man the innate ability to "tell time" (Genesis 1:14). Now prior to the creation of the Earth and the universal cosmos, there was just the Godhead in eternity. At some immeasurable point, They (the threeness of the Godhead) created celestial beings—nonillions of them. As the creative Father of this vast angelic host, the Godhead was recognized as the Father, the Word, and the Holy Spirit, all coequal in a holy, harmonious Oneness. There is no First, Second, or Third Person, as you may hear people say; I do not agree with that incorrect pronouncement, and you will find no statement like that anywhere in Scripture. The Father is God (Deuteronomy 32:6); the Word is God (John 1:1); and the Holy Spirit is God (Acts 5:3–4), Threeness-in-Oneness, and Oneness-in-Threeness! In fact, after the Word came to Earth to dwell in human form (John 1:14) for a specific purpose, He stated to a hostile religious group of Jewish Pharisees that "the Father and I are one" (John 10:30).

By the way, just to throw this out to you, the Godhead's "rest" in Genesis 2:2 was not the type of rest humans take upon becoming tired. The use of "rest" in that passage of Scripture is simply a metaphor for halted, stopped, or ceased (i.e., They had finished creating all that They desired), and then set the day after Their six-day creative endeavor as a type of "day of celebration" of the most massive building project imaginable. So that day of celebration, that seventh day, was made holy so that mankind may emulate God, rest from their six days of working, and celebrate with God by praising, honoring, and acknowledging Him for His awesome creation. It should be done via God-centered activities, not self-centered activities of worldly pleasure.

In all actuality, the Godhead never stops working; Jesus even said so Himself (John 5:17). The great thing about it that you will never, ever find in humans is the Godhead's unshakable, unbreakable holy unity; They are the epitome of DASA. The Godhead's "DASA" is stamped on the entirety of Scripture, from Genesis to Revelation. Before time began, the Godhead (Father, Word, and Holy Spirit) was a spiritual Entity (John 4:24). Scripture shows Them working in tandem both implicitly and explicitly. Look at this profound example: the Father spoke the word which created the universe. After that, with a focus on this planet, the Holy Spirit moved over the ocean's surface.

Now being in DASA mode, you would break Genesis 1:1–2 down like this: Together, the Godhead, in Their threeness, enacted creation; the Father spoke it, the Word did it, and the Holy Spirit energized (gave movement to) it. This activity is supported by Psalms 33:6, 9 and 148:5; and Hebrews 11:3. To be clear on the profundity of this, it will be puzzling or nebulous even to a saint, especially if he or she is prone to being controlled by human emotions. For this to make sense, you must be suited and booted in the word of God and tuned in DASA.

DASA (DYNAMIC APPLICATION OF SPIRITUAL AWARENESS)

Whether anyone, saints or unbelievers, becomes angry at me for boldly saying these things, well, it proves several points:

- You reject God like the Jewish Israelites did thousands of years ago (1 Samuel 8:7–8; Psalm 2:3; and Luke 10:16).
- You dislike me because I boldly and publicly share the truth of God's holy word (John 15:20).
- Jesus rightly accuses you of sin, so you hate Him without a cause and refuse to believe in Him (John 7:7; 15:18, 25; 16:9).

Nearly everyone who claims that the Bible "was tampered with," "is full of contradictions," or "is nothing but gobbledygook" are people who are disgruntled and love living the lifestyle that their father, the devil, has deceived them into accepting. Unbeknownst to the devil's followers, though, is that their temporary "pleasure" is not a lifestyle. It is a deathstyle, according to Proverbs 14:12 and Matthew 7:13. The problem with people who are doggedly determined and sinfully self-willed is that they will allow nothing, not even the Godhead, to stand in their way. It is similar to drug addicts crazed for "a fix." They will rob siblings, parents, relatives, close friends, or even kill just to get that "fix" their minds crave.

Satan is the "needle" that has injected the drug of delusion into the minds and hearts of his children so that they will crave the "pleasures" of this world-system and fight, steal, and kill to keep it. This is no different from what people several thousand years ago craved (Numbers 11:4–5; Psalm 78:18; John 8:44).

Multiple millions of people from practically every nation on the planet make this claim: "I love God." "I love the Lord." That may be truly stated, but it is not a statement of truth, and here is the reason why. They speak from a human, emotional viewpoint, and not according to DASA. It is indeed self-evident that they do not truly love God according to Luke 9:23 and John 14:15–16. This is one of the biggest problems with the masses of people; they want to "love" God their way, from rank human emotion, instead of God's way (Isaiah 56:6; Matthew 22:37; 1 John 3:18–19). With DASA, however, it allows you to dispense with limited finite emotions that shift and change like sand on a beach, and instead, provides you the spiritual awareness of Godhead-empowered stability (Colossians 2:9–10).

The Godhead in Subtleness

Practically everyone claiming to be a Christian is familiar with the terms Father, Son, and Holy Spirit. I dare say a good many do not fully comprehend the full implications of those titles. To get an idea of what I mean, if you have read, studied, practiced, and put DASA into motion steadfastly over the past sixty days or more, you are serious about Jesus, and I commend you. So do this: ask a Christian if he or she knows the name of the Father, the Son, and the Holy Spirit. Then wait for their response.

The way to determine if a person is speaking through human intellect or from a DASA standpoint lies in the answer he or she provides you. By the way, the question is sparked by the Scripture, Matthew 28:19. There is only one correct answer that may be expressed in several different ways: "Jesus!" "His name is Jesus." "It's Jesus." "The answer is Jesus." If they do not give you an answer like that or something similar, then it is more than likely they are trying to verbalize what they simply do not fully comprehend. I will give you three Scripture hints and let you use DASA to comprehend the answer (Acts 4:12; Philippians 2:9–11; Colossians 3:17).

As your DASA matures and is strengthened by perpetual usage, you will find that the Godhead communicates with you through the sword of the Spirit or through the Spirit Himself, as He did with two men in Acts 13:2. When the Godhead sees the strong desire in you to give Him first place in your life above all else, as stated in Psalm 37:4–5, Matthew 6:33, and Romans 12:1, He gives an ear to your communication (prayers, requests, and praises) and readily dialogues with you (2 Chronicles 7:14; Proverbs 15:8).

Here is something exciting you will probably notice happening: You will barely be able to read more than a few paragraphs in the word of God before He shows you a new revelation that you had not seen before, though you may have read that passage of Scripture

DASA (DYNAMIC APPLICATION OF SPIRITUAL AWARENESS)

many times previously. It is like having a storage silo filled to the rafters with treasures of every kind, and each time you excitedly dig through it, you continuously find sparkling new gems (Proverbs 2:4; Ephesians 3:8; Colossians 2:3).

What I believe the Holy Spirit wants me to share with you now is a little of something you never noticed, even though you may have read God's word for many years. When He began enlightening me on this, I was exceptionally surprised at how many there are. Even after eagerly and intently being studious in the word of truth for four, six, even eleven hours a day, and sometimes all night long and into the next day, doing this for over five years, even up to the point of authoring this book, I still look eagerly forward to studying and romping through this treasure trove of the Godhead (Hebrews 4:12). So get excited because you are going to truly enjoy what the Spirit of Truth is about to open up your mind to, that most likely compels you to desire more of this scriptural knowledge.

The actual word *Godhead* is used as a way to express the three-fold nature of one supreme Being who reveals Himself at will as one entity (Exodus 6:3), or as a tripartite entity (Mark 1:10–11). But even when He "separates" into three, They are still harmoniously and intrinsically linked. This profound explanation can be simply illustrated using something natural like a physical liquid. Consider this example: one single cup of H_2O can exist in three separate states: water, ice, or steam (vapor), and each of the three can revert back to that same single cup of H_2O. However, there aren't three waters; all three are unified within each other. That is essentially how it is with the Godhead—Threeness in Oneness, and Oneness in Threeness. Therefore, there is only one God we worship (Isaiah 43:10).

The word *Godhead* appears only twice in the Bible, especially in the Old King James Version and also the New King James Version. Although other versions may use a different word than *Godhead*, it does not detract from His tripartite nature. However, I personally prefer the word I use exclusively here—Godhead! The following will enlighten you on how They are always working in tandem, whether as Oneness or a seemingly separate Threeness (e.g., Jesus's comment in John 5:19). Additionally, the Three of Them live within a born again believer as just one Godhead Spirit.

There is one Godhead who, before Jesus's earthly ministry, was a combined Father, Word, and Holy Spirit. After the Word came to earth and took on the body of Jesus, He was called the Son of God, as shown in Psalm 2:7, Luke 1:26–35, Acts 13:32, and Hebrews 1:5. After Jesus's death, resurrection, and subsequent ascension to heaven, as explained in Acts 1:9–11, the Godhead became Father, Son, and Holy Spirit, which are His current titles. Now let us see this Oneness of the Godhead working as a harmonious holy team.

In Luke 1:35, you see the Holy Spirit, the Father (Most High), and the Son of God (Jesus) all intrinsically connected. About 30 years after that, another separated but harmoniously linked scene appears (Luke 3:21–22). The Godhead unity is shown in Romans 5:5–6 (God, the Holy Spirit, and Christ). Romans 8:9–10 should remove any confusion you may have. Look at how Paul connects the Godhead Members in Romans 15:16. Now go to Romans 15:30; Paul specifically mentions each Member of the Godhead. You see Jesus, the Holy Spirit, and God's unity in 1 Corinthians 2:2–5. Then in Galatians 3:14, God, through Jesus, blessed us to receive the Holy Spirit.

If you are a saint, then you are a product of the Godhead; when you believed in Christ, He gave you the Holy Spirit, who is God's guarantee of the inheritance saints will receive (Ephesians 1:13–14). Do you see from all this how the three members of the Godhead are perpetually operating in unified oneness? Again, Paul lists each member of the Godhead in Ephesians 4:4–5—one Spirit (the Holy Spirit), one Lord (Christ Jesus), and one God and Father. In an earlier chapter, you already discovered how Jesus is the embodiment of the entire Godhead (Colossians 2:9). In 1 Peter 1:2, God knew you, the Holy Spirit made you holy, as you were cleansed by the blood of Jesus; all of them working cohesively as one Godhead (Revelation 1:4–6). The only two places that word is found are Romans 1:20 and Colossians 2:9.

As I mentioned, the holy interrelation of members of the Godhead is rather explicit if you are in DASA mode as you study

62

DASA (DYNAMIC APPLICATION OF SPIRITUAL AWARENESS)

God's word. But those who live a lifestyle dictated by their human emotions are not able to comprehend this reality that is so numerous in the New Testament because it can only be discerned by the dynamic application of spiritual awareness (1 Corinthians 2:14). I have listed only a handful of the Godhead members' cohesiveness. As you study the four Gospels and the Epistles, I suggest you indicate in some way or other each time you discover a Scripture passage showing Them in action as One. Some are very subtly shown, but if your DASA is strong, you will find them. Here's an example for those who have read the word for years. Look how subtle this is; they pray to the Father for saints' hope in Jesus, powered by the Holy Spirit (1 Thessalonians 1:3–5).

I will give you one more group so that you may cogitate it through DASA:

1. Jesus, in John 2:19, said that He will raise Himself.
2. Romans 1:4 says it was the power of the Holy Spirit that raised Jesus.
3. But the power of the Father is the source for raising Jesus in Romans 6:4.

Happy cogitation!

God's Will

Starting with the Father Himself, He set the prime example for everyone else to follow. He did not carry out His own will to judge; instead, He let Jesus do the judging (John 5:22). Following that example, Jesus, unselfishly, did not carry out His own will but judged according to the Father's will (John 5:30), as He stated very plainly in John 6:38. And not to be outdone, the other Member of the Godhead followed suit; He did not speak on His own but only what He received from Jesus. Because of that holy, perfect example, we need to be DASA-tuned, *not doing* our will nor speaking what we want but only what we are told by the Godhead (Luke 9:23; 12:11; 1 John 3:23).

There are moments when one may become so overwhelmed with spiritual joy that it flows outward and is reflected by the physical emotion of tears, laughter, or a sense of satisfaction at pleasing the Lord, etc., but you are spiritually taught, not emotionally wrought. For example, I was praising and worshiping the Godhead with one of the many songs inspired by me by the Holy Spirit. As I was nearing the end of the song, I was so spiritually awestruck at the lyrical arrangement and melody, how beautifully it sounded, singing about each Member of the Godhead, that I just could not stop my tears from flowing. I began communicating with Him then, telling Him how much I appreciate this incredible joy He placed within me and thanking Him for allowing me to actually participate in composing sweet Christian songs of praise. Keep in mind, though, that this is DASA-controlled spirituality that positively impacts you.

Being in DASA mode brings one to the point where they eagerly look forward to doing the Godhead's will (Psalm 40:8; 1 Peter 4:2). With each Godhead member unashamedly deferring to the other's will, it creates a dynamic, unbreakable, harmoniously holy circle of respectfully honoring another. We must do likewise (Romans 12:10; Philippians 2:3). Jesus said you will not enter His kingdom if you refuse to do His will (Matthew 7:21). He also said you are His friend if you obey His command (John 15:14).

It is eternally detrimental to one's very soul to ignore the will and command of the Godhead. One of my most sincere prayers is that together we will touch many hearts so that they may see just how serious an infraction it is to neglect the Godhead's impassioned plea to come to the spiritual safety of His will and commands, especially regarding holiness. We touched on holiness in chapter 4, under the "Sanctified?" heading. However, the Holy Spirit feels it is critical to expand on it for your sake, so that no one who reads this will have any excuse on the day of judgment, saying they knew nothing about all of this, and no one ever explained it. So continue reading because it is a dreadful thing to fall into the hands of the living God (Hebrews 10:31).

The Godhead wants you to realize that holiness should be your burning, yearning desire (2 Corinthians 7:1) because He chose you

DASA (DYNAMIC APPLICATION OF SPIRITUAL AWARENESS)

to be holy even before the beginning of time (Ephesians 1:4). The Godhead works deep within you to help you have a strong desire to do what is pleasing to Him (Philippians 2:13). Keep in mind that unless you get a Bible and read and ponder each and every Scripture I list, none of the content of this book will have any significance. It is imperative to take the time to read and consider every Scripture reference as you arrive at them; there should be no hurry. If, for some reason, you are pressed for time, my suggestion is that you peruse this book during a time-favorable period more convenient to your edification. If you feel you don't need to read any of the listed Scriptures, then please close this book and continue in your secular lifestyle.

Understand and bury in your mind that it is the Godhead's will for you to be holy (1 Thessalonians 4:3). This is made even more relevant by Hebrews 10:10. Use this book as an aid to your Bible; it may be instrumental in equipping you to understand the spiritual dynamics of doing His will (Hebrews 13:21). As you make DASA your perpetual source, you need to actuate the word of God, not just read or listen to it. To solidify it all, one of the apostles in Jesus' "inner circle" of three said it very emphatically: "You must be holy" (1 Peter 1:15). Lastly, anyone who willfully refuses to abide by this is rejecting God Himself, as shown in 1 Thessalonians 4:8.

Christian Virtues

DASA trains and strengthens you to focus on the reality of being holy and rely on virtues that may positively impact the society around you, instilling peace and harmony. Although the myriad human-developed programs that attempt to guide people "on a straight path" in life are well-intended, they are merely finite, temporal, human ideas that do little to nothing in the way of enlightening people to the sinful nature of humanity and fall woefully short of bringing people's hearts to match spiritual integrity according to the word of God.

Human effort can never and will never restrain sinful human nature, which is contrary to a holy Godhead. Trying to live apart from the righteousness established by the Godhead blots out His holiness, making it impossible to have a personal relationship with Him and to have Jesus call you His friend (John 15:14). And unless you allow the Holy Spirit to lead your life, you are most certainly headed for eternal destruction (Matthew 7:13; 2 Thessalonians 1:9).

What's wrong with most of the world's educational leaders is that they implement constantly shifting ideas, steps, studies, plans, etc., for students or patients to follow. With this constant humanistic churning, people are hard-pressed to find sure footing, which leads them to the type of conclusive results they desperately seek. DASA, on the other hand, once implemented from requisite practice, puts you on a level far superior to the weak, temporal plans and programs of social and allopathic-medical educators. Being word-of-God-based, DASA sits unshakable, firm, on a permanent foundation (Matthew 7:24–25; Luke 16:17; Psalm 119:89).

Remember when we discussed the dialogue between Nicodemus and Jesus? Nicodemus was a highly educated, prominent leader among his peers who must have invested many years of study to rise to such a high position. Nevertheless, his education and high rank scored zero with Jesus, and Nicodemus could not comprehend even one of the basic truths of the Christian faith—being born again (John 3:10). So it is no wonder today's so-called MDs and PhDs who are educators cannot "get it right"; they have the Nicodemus syndrome! And the majority of them are worldly, indifferent, unbelievers, agnostics, or atheists.

DASA employs biblical-based virtues that are obviously distinct from the world's point of view, and Christ-followers operating in DASA mode are looked upon as weird (1 Peter 4:4). But the good thing is that we are not out to score points with them nor win their approval; we seek only to please our Lord and obtain rewards from Him (Matthew 5:11–12; 2 Corinthians 5:9; 1 Thessalonians 4:1; Hebrews 10:35).

The great thing about DASA mode is that it is powered by the spiritual might of the Holy Spirit Himself. As you glide along in this mode, seek the fruit He wants to produce in you: love, joy, peace, patience, kindness, goodness, faithfulness, gentleness, and self-control (Galatians 5:22). The surrounding society is not pre-

DASA (DYNAMIC APPLICATION OF SPIRITUAL AWARENESS)

pared for that; they will think you are freaked out of your mind. Some will mock you; others will deride you. But with the word-of-God ammunition loaded into your heart, your spiritual awareness fires off Matthew 5:11–12, applying it "at the moment" to the situation (i.e., dynamic application)! Almost immediately, another shot is fired (Matthew 5:44), and noticing how calm you are as you smile and remain joyful while exhibiting self-control, begins to freak *them out*! As your good deeds shine (Matthew 5:16), it gives you greater encouragement, allowing you to be strong, immovable, and working enthusiastically as mentioned in 1 Corinthians 15:58.

Because God was so loving to forgive us through Christ for a whole slew of sins, we need to be tenderhearted as well (Matthew 18:21–22; Ephesians 4:32). What Jesus did was break down to the bare essentials what everyone needs to know about spiritual guidance. DASA is instrumental in making you keenly aware of and applying that guidance knowledge. So filtering through DASA the virtues listed in Galatians 5:22, as well as more to follow, will help you transcend all the agony, pain, and suffering that various circumstances may potentially cause.

Millions of people the world over enjoy collecting things. You yourself may have a collection hobby: stamps, comic books, antique cars, rare coins. I used to have a collection of rocks I picked up from various countries I visited. I had a whole box of them and carried them around for many years. Stupid rocks! What in *rock nation* was I thinking? Who knows? Maybe I was the one freaked out of my own mind. Anyway, it was all for nothing. And when you multiply that action many times over, we have innumerable amounts of people collecting stuff. Eventually, it gets lost, tossed, traded, handed down, or in other cases, sold. Despite it all, however, it is still worldly, temporal junk in God's eyes (Matthew 6:19–21).

As you build yourself up in DASA, biblical virtues should be what you collect, in line with Matthew 6:21. They are invaluable as a collection for which God will commend you. So start focusing more on these "gems of heaven." Here are some you may add that is different from the previous: focus on what is true, honorable, right, pure, lovely, and admirable. Think about things that are excellent and worthy of praise (Philippians 4:8). Remember, all those virtues are intangible and deciphered through your mind, where your spiritual awareness may dynamically apply them as needed. Be a Scripture collector.

Our God, as you know, is the God of love—agape love (1 John 4:8). Love is intrinsic to His holiness, and the two qualities cannot be separated any more than light can be separated from the sun, or wetness from water, or a minute from time, or coldness from snow. And God's love is immeasurable, unfathomable (Romans 8:38–39). Jesus emphasized it in John 15:12, 17, and as you saw in Galatians 5:22, love is listed first among the spiritual fruits of the Holy Spirit. As you should have noticed, the Godhead is in action in the sentence before this. So is it any surprise that God would place love "above all" other virtues (Colossians 3:14)? In 1 Timothy 6:11, some virtues are repeated, and new ones are added.

All the virtues under the subheading "Christian Virtues" should be pursued with the tenacity of treasure hunters. Something to keep in mind is the old saying, "No man is an island." This means that even though your DASA is very strong, you cannot always do things alone. You need to *hang out* with Christ-followers; get recharged spiritually in godly conversations with them. We live in a very sinful world, and you will not be able to avoid associating with degenerate people (1 Corinthians 5:9–10). But as much as you possibly can, make associating with Christ-followers your top priority. Have godly fun together, like competing over who has collected the most virtues in their spiritual awareness.

Interesting Doubles

In some cases, some may not understand a particular Scripture and so may mark it as doublespeak or contradiction. Take a look at a few and see what you think:

- Jesus is the gate. He's the shepherd (John 10:7, 11).
- The Father testifies about Jesus. Jesus testifies about the Father (John 5:37; 17:6–8).

DASA (DYNAMIC APPLICATION OF SPIRITUAL AWARENESS)

- The Father allows access to Jesus. Jesus allows access to the Father (John 6:44; 14:6).
- God issued the breath of life in the beginning (Genesis 2:7).
- Jesus will issue the breath of death in the end (2 Thessalonians 2:8).
- God Almighty said, "I AM!" (Exodus 3:14).
- Jesus said, "I AM!" (John 8:58).
- Old body by God—terrestrial (Genesis 2:7); new body by God—celestial (2 Corinthians 5:1–5).
- The Spirit of God / the Spirit of Jesus (Genesis 1:2; Galatians 4:6).
- *An* angel of the Lord. *The* Angel of the Lord (Luke 2:9; Exodus 3:2).
- The Creator (Genesis 1:1) is the "Father" (Malachi 2:10); the Creator (Hebrews 1:10) is the "Everlasting Father" (Isaiah 9:6).

The word of God is replete with "interesting doubles" from Genesis to Revelation. Too many people simply "read" God's word without eagerness, enthusiasm, or true zeal. DASA practitioners, however, like chickens pecking at corn, pursue the word with gusto and ramped-up excitement. These are the ones who do not want to become spiritually drab. When you become seriously interested in studying it, instead of just reading it with no real interest, things will start to pop. Here is an example: When saints, or even those who ain't, read a passage like 2 Thessalonians 1:1, most of them derive practically nothing from the very first sentence. But in DASA mode, saints will see Silas's name and think, *Wow! Silas was not just some low-rank sidekick of Paul. He was a prominent church leader, teacher, prophet, and speaker from the Jerusalem Church* (Acts 15:22, 32, 35). Paul realized his true value when he chose Silas to accompany him on a missionary journey after Paul had contended with Barnabas over an issue (Acts 15:40). Together, as they traveled from place to place sharing the gospel, they were scorned, mocked, derided, belittled, beaten, chased out of town, stoned, jailed, and even had terrorist plots against Paul's life.

DASA mode, as I stated in a previous chapter, is perpetual. As you practice, there may be some *fumbling* initially. But once it is strengthened, you really won't have to pay much attention to it because it will settle on you in subtle ways, something like "set it and forget it." It will be so automatic you'll think it is natural, sort of like your eyes blinking throughout the day (i.e., a controlled natural response).

As you have already seen since reading up to this point, the word of God is a treasure trove of amazing Scriptures. It took me several years of being studious in the sword of the Spirit to match and group them in the way you have seen here. This should make it more convenient for you so that you don't have to hunt and scratch; it's all there for you, neat and conveniently *wrapped*. Perhaps you have appreciated being enlightened on the Godhead, the triune Creator of everything, both tangible and intangible. You may also have noticed my lack of use of popular terms like *Rapture* (the Rapture), *Trinity*, or *Saint* with the capital letter *S*, or other such terms tossed around in Christendom. I do not follow trends or things that become popular just because *everybody else* is saying or doing it. I only do this—stay in DASA mode and follow Christ as He said (Luke 9:23).

Before I close out this chapter, I would like to share a few more Scriptures with you that should help you as you endure your own trials, hardships, and tribulations while simultaneously sharing the gospel of Jesus Christ with others unashamedly (Romans 1:16). First of all, keep in mind this about the Godhead: He is just one, not three Gods, even though you see the usage of plural words in reference to Him (e.g., Us, Our, We, Their). Those words simply let us know that though He is truly one single eternal Entity, He has an intrinsically triune nature. And I will again use H_2O as an example so this profound information will be as clear to you as the air between this page and your eyes; H_2O has an intrinsic, triune nature:

- Take one pot of water; put it in the freezer.
- Soon, the water becomes solid ice.

DASA (DYNAMIC APPLICATION OF SPIRITUAL AWARENESS)

- Then take the pot of solid ice and place it on a heated surface; it soon manifests as water and continues to manifest as vapor over time.

Notice, then, that there are not three waters; it's one pot of water. There are not three blocks of ice; it's one solid block of ice. And there are not three vapors; it's one vapor from the one pot of water that manifested as one pot of ice—just one! They are all one and the same. This is a natural way to explain the Godhead's triune reality. He stamped that reality on the entire universe.

Apostle Paul made a statement in one of his letters indicating that what he was about to say was what God told him (e.g., Jeremiah 1:9, John 12:49). And he wanted to assure his readers that his writing came "directly from the Lord" (1 Thessalonians 4:15). But can that statement be substantiated? Well, look at Acts 9:3–6. Quite some years after that, Paul had another experience that relatively few other servants of God had; Isaiah had it (Isaiah 6:1–4); Stephen had it (Acts 7:55–56); and also the Apostle John had it (Revelation 1:1–2). However, Paul did not want to make his readers feel as though he was boasting in any way (2 Corinthians 12:1–5). And in Galatians 1:15–17, Paul states how God had predetermined all this for him even before he was born.

Again, something regarding what Apostle Paul stated should be expounded upon and made crystal clear to this modern-day generation of people because some denominations within Christianity, that are well-meaning but misinformed, are causing many believers to be misdirected and in spiritual bondage, which impacts them physically as well. Paul alluded to the fact that, when our spirits are not with the body, our spirits are present with the Lord in heaven. You will see this in 2 Corinthians 5:1–8.

Now if someone tells you that he or she longs for something or to be somewhere, that means there are no intermediates or exceptions. And that is exactly what Paul meant in Philippians 1:23. He knew if he were to die that very day, his body would be buried here on earth, but his spirit would be escorted immediately to heaven to be in the presence of Christ Jesus, as exemplified in Luke 23:43. Some denominations will have you believe in some sort of "soul sleep" where your spirit, soul, and body lie dormant in the grave until everyone on the planet is resurrected on the "last day." This type of teaching is clearly in error. Christian leaders may be subjected to the consequences described in 1 Corinthians 3:15 for this erroneous teaching.

Christ-followers alone are the ones the Lord Jesus will call up to Him in the clouds, both the ones who have died and the living, according to 1 Thessalonians 4:14–18. Paul did not fabricate those words or that scenario; he was speaking exactly what Jesus told him to relay to other saints. Everyone else who is not a saint will not be included; they will be left in a world, this earth, that will go through seven years of horrific evil unimaginable in the minds of human beings (Matthew 24:21–22). Again, only those who reject the following will in no way possibly ever see the kingdom of God or experience the eternal presence of Christ:

- Matthew 16:24–26; Luke 14:27
- John 1:12
- Romans 3:22; 10:9–10; 12:1–2
- 1 Corinthians 6:18

The Scriptures prove that no Luke 9:23 Christ-followers will be judged by the Lord Jesus Christ for sins (Romans 5:9; 8:1; Ephesians 4:30). And since being with Christ means eternal existence, death is the opposite of that. Eternal life (John 3:15) connotes perpetual living with God. Eternal death implies perpetual dying; that is, it has no finality, unlike those teaching in error would lead you to believe. They teach that it (death in sin) is an end in itself. Jesus Himself, in His illustration of the rich man and Lazarus, shows us there is no end in itself but suffering forever (Luke 16:19–31). Those teaching in error try to tap into your emotions by using the rationalization that an Almighty, all-loving God would not torture someone for all eternity. What they are really doing is attempting to apply human logic to God's way of justice. And that is where they are in error (Isaiah 5:16; Hebrews 1:8) because they try pulling the Godhead down to their level of understanding, which is ludicrous (Isaiah 55:8–9).

Chapter 9

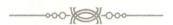

Food from the Godhead

Our forefathers, thinkers, businesspeople, and inventors, perpetually worked toward improvement in varied and myriad things to make this world a potentially "better place to live." Technically speaking, the world is a better place in terms of rapid transportation (automobiles, public vehicles like buses, trains/subways, and airplanes); there are all-in-one homes (living rooms, dining rooms, bedrooms, kitchens, bathrooms, and many with car space or attached garages). There are apartment buildings within close proximity to metropolitan areas to facilitate easy access to workplaces, as well as superhighways providing convenient travel to faraway areas within nations.

Food planting, harvesting, processing, producing, packaging, and transporting are amazingly quick, and able to be preserved over long periods: weeks, months, and even years for some perishables and other foods. It is also exceptionally easy to obtain via corner neighborhood markets, local farmers' markets, delicatessens, supermarkets, warehouse stores, and massive superstores. Additionally, there is a dizzying array of utensils and small machinery to make food preparation and cooking a convenience in the home. Unfortunately, there is a downside to all the technological advancements. It is tantamount to the euphemism, "collateral damage," where much of the nutritional value inherent in plant life the Godhead created on the third day is destroyed for the sake of speed.

The Godhead knew exactly what He was doing in creating food that provides exceptional nutrition to each and every one of the multiple billions of cells that sustain these terrestrial bodies which He created with intent and purpose. For the last two days of His creative process, days five and six, God had completed in abundance all that was necessary for a vibrant existence that was illness- and disease-free. Looking back, notice how, on day three of creation, He separated water and land so the land could become dry and get both sunshine and air. Afterward, He spoke to the land, and the power of His word brought forth endless varieties of plants, herbs, and fruit trees, all with the ability of self-replication (Genesis 1:11–13). The power of God's word to accomplish His purpose is told in Isaiah 55:11.

With the sea separated from the land, the Godhead filled the waters with a dizzying assortment of innumerable sea life. The Almighty Master Craftsman finalized creation, first with myriad living creatures both massively large and infinitesimally tiny (e.g., germs). Lastly, His "masterpiece" was made in His own image, with His characteristics. Think about it this way: during a female's pregnancy, on many occasions, everything possible is prepared in advance of the forthcoming masterpiece—a baby in your image. You ensure all is ready: crib, sheets, blankets, clothing, socks, booties, diapers, wet wipes, etc. Is it any wonder that God did it for us (Genesis 1:3–25)?

For the most part, mankind has depleted the world's food supply of much of the nutritional quality God created innately within it. Attempting to imitate God, mankind fortifies foods and drinks with *pick 'n' choose* vitamins and/or minerals, much of it is low-grade chemical reproductions or isolated "active" elements of various plants and herbs. It is sheer lunacy when they isolate a single "active" element from the hundreds that God placed within, just so they may patent it, neologize it, and market it at inflated prices. Renowned herbalist, Paul Schulick, lets us know that, contrary to isolating constituents from their source, those sources (plants, fruits, herbs) consist of an infinitely complex, God-supplied array of elements. What you should know is that when an organic source is eaten, as it is absorbed into your system a therapeutic effect is created as the hun-

DASA (DYNAMIC APPLICATION OF SPIRITUAL AWARENESS)

dreds of elements produce synergism; this is what God intended as alluded to in Genesis 1:29.

Alas, despite all that God has abundantly provided, and regardless of the incredible advances in technology by humanity that make the world a *better place to live*, there is one thing that cancels it all out (Genesis 6:5; Jeremiah 17:9; Matthew 15:19). And rather than to adhere to Proverbs 3:5, humans trust in their own, wicked heart, refusing to plant and harvest as God commanded (Leviticus 25:1–7). It is this stiff-neck refusal that we have poor quality plants in this current day and age. We plant and harvest in never-ending cycles, giving the land no rest, which depletes the nutritional value whereby plants are imbued. Moreover, vegetation and trees are sprayed with chemical toxins that negatively impact the quality of what little nutritional value remains. Adding even further to this mess are the dyes and wax used on plants to make them appear more brightly colored or shiny. The juices of plants and fruits are reduced to nothing more than flavored drinks when they are stripped of their powerful nutritional essence through mankind's pasteurization process with subsequent *fortifying* it with minimal, selected pharmaceutical *vitamins*.

Interestingly, advanced technology is also used in nefariously financial ways (i.e., processing food at speeds geared to the fastest most efficient delivery methods to masses of people), sacrificing high quality for high speed. With their minds mainly on profit margins, simply passing USDA grading standards at the lowest levels of inspection suffices in this industry. Mass marketers package food with brightly colored, highly illustrated pictures of fruits and vegetables, but this blinds the minds of unwary purchasers. And prices are lowered to the point of nutritionally inferior food being favored over organics bursting with high-level nutritional constituents.

Though taking a little more time to come to market, organics are handled with a greater level of care and are not subject to being sprayed with toxic chemicals such as chlorinated hydrocarbons, mercury compounds, fumigants, and fungicides.

Do not be deceived by the marketing sophistry of mass marketers. In any case, you would be better off supplementing each meal with certified organic multivitamins or a "whole-food-based" multivitamin. This ensures your body is well-supplied with the highest caliber of nutrients it was created to receive. Price-wise, it may seem too expensive, as many shoppers believe. Okay, let's compare their medical or pharmaceutical prescription bill to a bottle of vitamins or their chemotherapy treatment by an allopathic doctor to the naturopathic treatment by an ND.

With an eye on the dollar sign more than on patients' total health, allopathic surgeons are more inclined to remove women's God-given breasts or surgically mutilate patients in feigned attempts to *root out cancer*. Be advised, more surgeries are hardly the answer. All too many surgeries are performed due to misdiagnosis and cause more harm than good. In fact, a study published in the allopathic medical profession's prestigious publication, the *Journal of the American Medical Association* (*JAMA*), by Dr. John Wasson, concluded that "we have, in essence, an epidemic of treatment and no scientific proof that it is valid. The take-home message is that we [MDs] don't know what we're doing, but we're doing a lot of it." That is a factual truth the allopathic medical profession keeps away from their patients. According to figures cited in JAMA, up to 140,000 patients die annually from adverse reactions to prescription drugs.[6,7]

Whether or not you agree, nearly all of the nation's illnesses and diseases stem from two realities; one is physical, and the other is spiritual:

1. Physically, the National Research Council concluded that the American diet was "probably the greatest single factor in the epidemic of cancer, particularly for cancers of the breast, colon, and prostate."
2. Spiritually, the word of God warned that ignoring, being disobedient to, or deviating from His truth brings horrific consequences (Deuteronomy 28:59–61).

---

[6] Classen, D.C., et al. *JAMA* 226, no. 20 (Nov. 1991)
[7] National Research Council, 1982. "Diet, Nutrition, and Cancer." Washington D.C.: National Academy Press, 55

DASA (DYNAMIC APPLICATION OF SPIRITUAL AWARENESS)

American processed food is permeated with about three thousand food additives, half of which make up people's diets. I am going to enlighten you about some processed *food*, (e.g., bologna, hot dogs [beef and chicken franks included], sausages, and canned soup). But first, take a look at some troubling statements by some of the allopathic medical profession's own prominent colleagues, physicians who were not parsimonious with their medical thoughts; they corroborate Dr. Wasson's published study in *JAMA*, which leads us to believe that curing illness and disease is not a high priority, yet they use incessant media sophistry to make you think otherwise and gain your trust. But notice the unadulterated truth:

> Unfortunately, there are more profits to be made in treating disease than in promoting prevention. (Kenneth H. Cooper, MD, MPH)

> If you're feeling well, just stay away from the doctor. (Eugene Robbins, MD, Professor Emeritus, Stanford University)

> The scientific basis of medicine is much weaker than most patients or even physicians realize; this leads to treatment based on uncertainty. (C. Everett Koop, MD, Former U.S. Surgeon General)

> We don't know what we're doing in medicine. Perhaps one-quarter to one-third of medical services…little or no benefit to patients. (Dr. David Eddy, Former Director, Duke University, Health Policy Research)

> The American public does not have the knowledge to make wise health-care decisions… Trust us. We will tell you what's good for you.

ADYM DANTZ

(David Kessler, Former FDA Commissioner on
Larry King Live, 1992)

Upon completing the reading of this chapter, you will have
added to your knowledge base and be equipped to make much better,
informed decisions for your personal health, or your family's health,
than what your allopathic doctor gives you credit for, and contrary
to what they assert.

Both prevention and cure are realities that the combined greed
of the medical profession, the pharmaceutical industry, and the FDA
go to great lengths to hide from you. Bear in mind, they do not want
you to know the truth that copious research points out, for example,
the terrible feeling of a cold's symptoms is potentially lengthened
in duration by either over-the-counter or prescriptive non-steroidal
anti-inflammatory drugs (NSAIDs). Even worse is that renal pelvic
cancer may be an adverse side effect for both men and women with
continued use of NSAIDs. It is because of the above truth, as well as
allopathic doctors' partiality to adverse-effect-riddled pharmaceutical drugs that I strongly urge DASA practitioners to first seek treatment from a naturopathic physician (N.D.) and follow his or her
recommendation(s).

Now let's move on with the undeniable truth about hot dogs
and other highly processed *food*. My Christian friend, who likes
to be called Solo, previously worked for over a decade in various
meat-packing and processing centers and served in various opera-
tional capacities. In a single workday, Solo viewed what the average
person does not see even in a lifetime. As he relayed to me his operation of the machinery used in the slaughtering and processing of
hundreds of bovines day and night, 1 Kings 8:63 comes to mind.

Without going into the great amount of detail it would take to
inform you of all that is involved in this revulsively gory operation,
I'll just share with you the pertinent information you should know
about the chemical-laden, sodium-saturated bologna, hot dogs, sausage, and canned soup you so lusciously chow down on often. Here
is one term you should never, ever forget: *pink slime*. The next time
you are oh so ready to wrap your lips around the "great American hot

DASA (DYNAMIC APPLICATION OF SPIRITUAL AWARENESS)

dog," you decorate with your favorite condiments, try looking at the wrapping it came in from the store; notice in the ingredients area, the word *by-product*. That word is actually a euphemism for, guess what, none other than *pink slime*, which is a gross mixture of parts of the animal you never get to see nor would you want to see. Hint: think *Fear Factor*. Pink slime is the end result of another term in the meat processing industry.

Chubs is the industry term for parts of the animal that never come to market for public view: eyelids, eyeballs, mucus membranes, veins, etc.—need I go on? They do not throw out these disgusting animal body parts. Instead, they grind them into a mush, much like the food in your mouth after you've chewed it up before swallowing, and with the blood, fat, and chemical additives, they churn out that *pink slime* which becomes what you have been conditioned to love: hot dogs, beef franks, chicken franks, bologna, sausage, and the cheap, 45 percent hamburger meat you purchase to make meatloaf, meat sauce, meatballs, or hamburger patties (actually, you should call them *hamburger fatties*). Obviously, this industry wastes nothing. The base for canned soup is the nasty stomach contents squeezed out of the dead animal, including the yellowish bile. Is it any wonder why this industry saturates that mess they call *food* with so many chemical additives? Well, that's enough about *Fear Factor*–type food. How about we now take a look at nutrition from Almighty God?

Healing Foods

Unknown to many people is the fact that the Almighty (Revelation 1:8), who created us from the ground, also provided within plants from the ground the ability to sustain us, prevent illness, and provide healing should illness breach our body's defenses. Studying God's holy Word of truth also contributes immensely to both your spiritual and physical well-being, as shown in Exodus 15:26, Psalms 103:3 and 107:20, and Proverbs 3:7–8. Jesus made it crystal clear when He commanded that we not live on just food but also by every Word He spoke because His Word is life (Matthew 4:4; John 6:27) and in John 6:63, He said His Word is life.

Just as the cosmetic industry has enslaved females to their products, the pharmaceutical industry has done likewise in enslaving gullible people to pharmaceutical drugs, both over-the-counter NSAIDs and prescription drugs. James 5:1–6 prophetically alludes to the billionaire Sackler family, owners of the, now bankrupt, Purdue Pharmaceutical company, who were slapped with a six-billion-dollar fine by the US Supreme Court. They intentionally misled allopathic medical physicians by training Purdue sales reps to lie to them by claiming that OxyContin was less addictive than some of the more popular prescription opioids.

Going on the notion it was a *long-acting* (i.e., time-release version of the addictive prescription narcotic, oxycodone), Purdue launched a 1996 multifaceted campaign which downplayed OxyContin's adverse effects. Justice Department investigative correspondence, however, proved that as early as 1999, Purdue knew that physicians were putting prescriptions on the market to Oxy abusers who gained quick "highs" by crushing the opioid into powder and snorting it. Interestingly, Purdue hired a former FDA-approving authority, who falsely claimed the safety of OxyContin, and doubled his FDA salary. It should not be surprising that approximately one-third of the American population is ingesting about eight or more doctor-prescribed drugs daily by age fifty. It is rare that an allopathic doctor (MD) would refer you to a naturopathic doctor (ND) to be treated with organic substances, nor would they simply tell you to eat a small handful of almonds to dissolve a headache.

DASA practitioners should always keep natural organic substances in their homes, as these provide both preventive healing and countermeasures against a variety of airborne, waterborne, and food-borne particles that may potentially cause bacterial, fungal, parasitic, or viral infections that negatively impact the proper functioning of your digestive, cardiovascular, respiratory, reproductive, and immune systems, as well as other vital internal organs. Pay close attention now, DASA practitioner; if your immune system is breached, the invading microorganisms overpower and weaken it, leaving you susceptible to symptoms of various illnesses and diseases. So let's take a look at several absolute organic must-haves.

DASA (DYNAMIC APPLICATION OF SPIRITUAL AWARENESS)

Almonds

Many enjoy almonds as a snack food, almond slivers added to salads, "almond chicken" at Chinese restaurants, almond "butter" as a much healthier alternative to peanut butter, and even almond milk, which is much better and healthier for human consumption than the casein in cow's milk. Almonds rank among the highest-protein nuts and are vital defenders against oxidative damage. Eating them on a daily basis makes you a less likely candidate for heart disease. Don't forget what I mentioned earlier about dissolving a headache with a small handful of almonds. The best thing about it all is that there are zero negative side effects.

Walnuts

Want a good night's rest every single night for the *rest* of your life? You cannot accomplish that long-term using OTC meds without being subject to adverse side effects. However, walnuts are naturally rich in God-supplied melatonin, encouraging a healthful sleep cycle. That's just a fraction of this superfood's true power. Walnuts are considered a high-end nut containing phytonutrients and antioxidants known to be helpful in reducing inflammation levels and warding off type 2 diabetes. Walnut's stellar reputation shines forth from its content of essential fatty acids such as alpha-linolenic and linoleic. As an excellent source of omega-3, even a four-ounce serving of salmon cannot match the nearly 100 percent of the total recommended omega-3 fatty acid intake you get from just a quarter cup of walnuts, with only 163 calories.

Honey

Unfortunately, all too many people are duped by commercial manufacturers that strip natural honey of much of its nutritional essence by cooking, diluting, filtering, and other processing methods, and then marketing it rather cheaply. At that point, it becomes nothing more than non-nourishing liquid sugar. Combined, Big

Pharma, medical allopaths, and the FDA's multibillion-dollar annual revenue stemming from the 800 percent markup on pharmaceutical drugs, from which exorbitant wealth is derived, makes them partial to these adverse-effect-riddled meds, to the detriment of honey— God's organic *medicine*.

Myriad extensive studies conducted on organic honey over several decades have identified the broad spectrum of all-natural medical attributes of honey. Though shunned, for the most part, by allopathic doctors (MDs), it is well-known within the naturopathic medical community that raw, organic, uncooked, undiluted, unfiltered honey delivers effectively the therapeutic values of herbs like ginger, while unleashing its own range of exceptional synergistic values. Allow me to enlighten you; eating honey activates within you many beneficial properties including antibacterial, anticancer, antifungal, antiulcer, and wound-healing effects. Imagine how many prescription meds it would take for all of that. And the cost? It is one of the factors that keep your bank account low. As a DASA practitioner, cogitate how the Godhead infused healing power into plant life and food sources like honey (Psalm 81:16; Proverbs 24:13; Isaiah 7:15). Did you know that your gastric mucosa can be protected by honey? With that reality, think of the potential cancer and ulcer eradication.

If possible, attempt to ascertain whether the honey you desire to purchase has been certified through any of the various state or international organizations such as OVON, OCIA, or Where Food Comes From Organic.

Lemons

Almighty God Himself, rather than scaring the heebie-jeebies out of us with His planet-shaking, mountain-crumbling voice as He did to the people in Exodus 20:18–19, chose to speak to us via the voices of human prophets He personally chose (Hebrews 1:1; 2 Peter 1:20–21). Upon completion of that, He Himself veiled His glory in a human body (Jesus) to speak to humanity from a human perspective (Deuteronomy 18:18–19; John 1:14). Sometimes, people do not always believe the truth when they read it (e.g., Psalm 33:6, 9). So

DASA (DYNAMIC APPLICATION OF SPIRITUAL AWARENESS)

Jesus demonstrated a fraction of the power of His spoken word as shown in the following: (1) Matthew 21:18–19; (2) Mark 4:35–41; and (3) John 11:43–44.

I had to share that with you so that you will know the truth of the unimaginable power the Lord can speak into anything or anyone. This brings us to lemons. God spoke so much healing power into the lemon fruit that it defies all human comprehension; lemons could almost be looked at as a mini-pharmacy within a fruit, but just without the adverse side effects and expense of prescription meds that allopathic doctors so readily give you. The legalized drug pushers, a.k.a. the pharmaceutical industry, would hate for stellar, truthful information such as this to reach the masses. But as a practitioner of DASA, I have faith that you will joyfully share this beneficial information among your family and friends, and also to your colleagues.

Let's take a look at some of the myriad health benefits of the neglected lemon; actually, let's just do seven of them:

- antibacterial
- antiviral
- contains immune-boosting power
- digestive aid
- helps in weight loss
- cleans your liver
- it's even a mosquito repellent

And as per results reported in a study by the *Annals of the Rheumatic Diseases*, lemons provide protection against inflammatory polyarthritis and osteoarthritis.

Untold millions of people suffer abject spiritual destitution because they willfully choose to neglect the only thing that can save them—the word of God (Hosea 4:6; John 6:63). Likewise, there are a tremendous number of people suffering needless illness and disease, simply from a lack of the type of knowledge you are now receiving about God's healing food sources. As you practice the dynamic application of spiritual awareness, you will be enlightened both spiritually and physically, which will be instrumental in precluding various maladies.

What I have shared with you about lemons are health facts by well-known naturopathic doctors (ND) but severely downplayed and ignored by allopathic doctors (MD). Nevertheless, you will be amazed by the exceptional power of additional benefits God spoke into this small yellow fruit that is highly effective against canker sores, corns and calluses, eczema, fatigue, high blood pressure, kidney stones, sore throat, and chills and fever of a cold, burns, and toothache, and it also freshens your breath. Good luck trying to get from an allopathic doctor just one single, non-bank-breaking prescription drug that can effectively treat all the above maladies with absolutely zero adverse side effects.

Ginger

If the people currently living in this world were not blinded by the neologistic sophistry of the pharmaceutical industry and the parsimonious medical thoughts of allopathic physicians, they could realize that ginger is truly an amazing wonder root. Ginger is among the superfoods of the world, and its effect on myriad symptoms of illnesses is nothing short of astonishing. Information about the medicinal properties inherent in ginger could fill several books, and all that I share with you here is only a summary. One of the most important things you need to know is that the National Cancer Institute (NCI) identified ginger among thirty-five other plant-based foods to be effective in preventing cancer (August 18, 2011, National Institute of Health [NIH] [.gov]).[8]

How can information as valuable as that be ignored in an America that is rife with cancer illness and much death from it? Why? I'll tell you why. Because the pharmaceutical industry uses its influence and multiple millions of dollars in advertising their adverse-effect-riddled drugs on thousands of large billboards across the country, splashed on full-page, colorful magazine advertisements, and on the most

---

[8]   http://www.ncbi.nlm.nih.gov>articles>PMC3426621

DASA (DYNAMIC APPLICATION OF SPIRITUAL AWARENESS)

watched *god* of this world—the television. But I hope we can form a *grassroot* informational word-of-mouth channel to let people know that ginger is indeed, and in essence, God's anticancer secret that has been revealed to His saints (Deuteronomy 29:29; Psalm 25:14).

Here is information that corroborates the NCI's proclamation. Research published in the *British Journal of Nutrition* has demonstrated the in vitro and in vivo anti-cancer activity of ginger, suggesting it may be effective in the management of prostate cancer. Other research shows the antitumor activity of ginger that may help defeat difficult-to-treat types of cancer, including lung, ovarian, colon, breast, skin, and pancreatic. Furthermore, because ginger helps prevent the toxic effects of many substances (including cancer drugs), it may be useful to ingest in addition to conventional cancer treatments.

For various pain relief, allopathic doctors will ask you, "What is your level of pain on a scale of one to ten?" Their sole purpose in asking you this is because there are specific NSAIDs corresponding to the numbers; the lower the number, the milder the medication; the higher the number, the stronger the medication. You really need to bear in mind that the more meds an MD has patients on, the better their incentives from the pharmaceutical companies.

On the "other side of the fence," NDs will be honest and upfront in telling you that ginger is better at relieving pain than ulcer-causing NSAIDs. These holistic physicians will advise you on the numerous, valuable, side effect-free health benefits of ginger, namely:

- supports healthy digestion, offering greater protein-digesting power than papaya
- soothes digestion
- contains at least twelve antiaging constituents that inactivate free radicals
- eases joint pain and fights internal infection as well as external sores
- twenty-two known constituents inhibit inflammatory 5-lipoxygenase, supporting prostate health

Do not think for even a second that Almighty God created ginger solely as a simple spice to enhance the flavor of foods, soften meat, and use for making tea. It is not considered a superfood for nothing. Guess what else is so magnificent about ginger? God made it to be both an all-natural preventative and curative. You think *that's* something? Consider all of the following:

- protects against Alzheimer's disease
- protects against ulcers
- protects the liver
- prevents duodenal and gastric disorders
- fights infections
- improves brain function
- counters both constipation and diarrhea
- strengthens your heart
- mitigates a female's menstrual cramp pains
- lowers blood sugar
- lowers cholesterol levels
- reduces soreness of muscles
- is anti-asthmatic
- antibacterial (i.e., inhibits toxic bacteria while promoting friendly species)
- is antifungal
- a potent anti-inflammatory
- antioxidant
- antiparasitic
- antiviral

All of what you see above is an undeniable truth that 99 percent of the allopathic physicians and surgeons in America will not disclose to you. But listen very carefully. There was a well-known group called the Eclectics. And no, I'm not referring to any 1960s singing group. The Eclectics was a prominent national group of more than twenty-five thousand American doctors who praised ginger, with many of them prescribing ginger to patients while noting ginger's sustained

DASA (DYNAMIC APPLICATION OF SPIRITUAL AWARENESS)

effects as an anti-inflammatory, systemic regulator, and body circulatory system tonic.

Listen, neither you nor I gain anything by me lying to you. In fact, all that I share with you about ginger is explicitly and exclusively detailed in *Ginger: Common Spice and Wonder Drug* by renowned herbalist, Paul Schulick. Factual, decades-long studies on the supreme effectiveness of ginger as compared to adverse-effect-riddled prescription drugs are truthfully presented to you along with charts, graphs, and statements from luminaries like former First Lady, Hillary Clinton; former US Court of Appeals, Seventh Circuit judge, Judge Cudahy; Dr. Claude Lenfant, former Director of the National Heart, Lung, and Blood Institute; and many others who agree that "it is painfully obvious our national health system is chronically ill—not to mention a very bad investment," says Paul Schulick.

As a DASA practitioner who is serious about being strengthened spiritually on a continual basis, and becoming an illness-resistant and potentially disease-free child of God (Deuteronomy 7:15; Psalm 103:3; Matthew 4:23), you need to ponder all of what you are being given insight into here; also do your best to internalize this invaluable knowledge the allopathic medical practitioners want to keep hidden from you.

With such proven healing power intrinsic to ginger, everyone, especially all DASA practitioners, should make it a top priority to keep plenty of ginger in the kitchen pantry at all times. It is truly a *God-created substance* that can guard you and your family's precious health 24-7. Trust God, ginger is one of the very best organic *medicines* you may invest in. The return on investment (ROI) health-wise is unsurpassed.

Body Pollution Solution

By allusion, we believe Almighty God actually spoke healing energy into His created food sources (Genesis 1:11–12; Psalm 33:3, 9). I have taken three of them—honey, lemons, and ginger—to create a bodily pollution solution, which I have dubbed Potent Trio.

With the Holy Spirit empowering you, the word of God instructing you, your DASA-breathing oxygenating your entire body and keeping you calm, as your emotions are kept in check, your dynamic application of spiritual awareness may help you produce much *fruit* as you go about activities and work for the kingdom of God. Unfortunately, because of a multiplicity of factors in this current world—bad eating habits, air pollution, water pollution, processed, chemically laced, GMO-produced foods, and other things that negatively impact our food supply—our physical bodies suffer nutritionally, resulting in potential physical illness.

Despite the adverse conditions above, the Potent Trio may preclude you from succumbing to the negative forces listed. Bodily ailments such as headaches, cold/flu, so-called heartburn, stomachaches, muscle cramps, dehydration, sore muscles, indigestion, and other energy-impeding symptoms can tax your mental and physical well-being, which may hinder your DASA practice as well. This would then be a situation where "the spirit is willing, but the flesh is weak" (Matthew 26:41).

In introducing the Potent Trio, I am not referring to King David's top three elite commanders in 1 Chronicles 11:11, where Jashobeam, the leader of the trio, fought three hundred enemy soldiers with his spear and killed them all in one single battle. What I am alluding to is one of the most potent, all-natural, sickness-defeating, disease-stopping, health-enhancing drinks probably ever unheard of. The reason why is that it is one of my own special, undiluted, powerful, organic drink formulations I concocted myself. Instead of producing it and marketing it for profit, though, that would not be Christ-like. My Lord and Savior wants me to help people by giving freely (Proverbs 21:26; Acts 20:35), so I freely give it. This DASA pollution solution will prevent the myriad germs breathed into and ingested into our bodies every second from taking a foothold. I have been using it for myself for many years now to keep my internal organs viral and bacteria-free and to keep my children cold-free, flu-free, and illness-free.

DASA (DYNAMIC APPLICATION OF SPIRITUAL AWARENESS)

The reason I also call it the Potent Trio is because it consists of honey, ginger, and lemons. Here is how to prepare it:

- Slice ginger into thin or thick slices, place into a small pot and add just enough water to cover the slices. Place on the stove and bring it to a boil. Then immediately turn it to a low setting so that it lightly simmers. Place a vented top on it and let it simmer for twenty minutes.
- While the ginger is simmering, take three to five lemons, slice each in half, and use a juice squeezer to squeeze them, including the pulp. Keep the seeds to plant or give away. Once you are finished, cover the lemon juice and set it aside. Once the twenty minutes are up on the simmering ginger, remove the pot to an unused burner, and let it sit until mildly warm (about two hours), but stir it about every half hour to encourage more juice content from the ginger.
- Once the ginger liquid is finger-touch warm, pour it, including the ginger slices, and the lemon juice into a large container. Then add the honey to your desired sweetness. Add more water if necessary to adjust the strength of the drink.

And voilà! There's your Potent Trio, DASA Pollution Solution. Now if you are by yourself, grab an eight or sixteen-ounce cup, pour in the Potent Trio, and sip on it while reading some Scriptures, relaxing in a comfy chair, or while listening to some Christian praise music. If family or company is there, pour them all a drink. As for me, I drink a cup several times a day every day, and it has been decades since I have had a headache, cold, flu, or any other viral or bacterial illness. You may either keep the container out at room temperature or put it in the fridge for a refreshing, ice-cold, delicious, health-enhancing drink.

With this Godhead-endorsed combination, no germ will dare attempt to invade your body. The Potent Trio puts bacteria, parasites, viruses, and any other germ on notice with "Warning! This body is off-limits." The organic honey, ginger, and lemons are able to stand on their own merits, like Jashobeam, the elite commander in 1 Chronicles 11:11, in terms of the ability of each one to assist your body's immune system in attacking and obliterating sickness-causing foreign invaders. But together, they are indeed an exceptional powerhouse, a formidable team, and a force to be reckoned with, just like the top three elite commanders, Jashobeam, Eleazar, and Shammah (2 Samuel 23:8–12).

It goes without saying that the DASA pollution solution is more than enough to hold its own. Coming from the Creator, though, He inundates His children with the best, abundantly (Malachi 3:10; 2 Corinthians 9:8). If you are constantly on the go, however, the second-best thing to do is to obtain powdered ginger in soft capsules (preferably 500 milligrams each) and take four or six of them with any drinks, snacks, or meals several times a day daily; the liquid gel extract soft capsules are fine also. Now with the Potent Trio arsenal guarding your circulatory system, that in itself is enough. But just to show you that our Lord wants you to be really healthy, check out the sheer power of a few more.

Coconut Oil

Hundreds of dollars are wasted by people every year simply by neglecting or having a lack of knowledge about, the health benefits of and the manifold uses of this superlative oil created by the Godhead for both your health and protection. Just to give you a glimpse, this amazing wonder oil may be used in your bathwater, as a lotion, as a massage oil, for dandruff control, as cooking oil, as furniture polish, and so much more. Just this one oil alone replaces all of the above, so you can see from just that how significant saving money could be. Of course, it would be best to obtain 100 percent virgin coconut oil. And take this into consideration: coconut oil provides a multitude of health benefits for your body, so wouldn't it make more sense to use a tablespoon of coconut oil rather than mineral oil for any bowel movement (constipation) problems? How about as an all-natural deodorant? Obtain *The Book on Internal STRESS Release*, which shows you not only how to use 100 percent virgin coconut oil

DASA (DYNAMIC APPLICATION OF SPIRITUAL AWARENESS)

as a deodorant but for more than twenty-five other things as well. Only a kind, compassionate, thoughtful, loving God would have the forethought to have planned all of that from the beginning of time. One of my favorite dishes is Chinese chicken fried rice. They cook it rather greasy though. So I'll prepare it at home using coconut oil, chopped chicken, salted fish, carrots, peas, and onions. It's a delicious, nutritious meal that can't be beaten.

Moringa Tree

Leaving off with fish, there are quite a few varieties: bass, mackerel, salmon, sardines, milkfish, trout, tuna, and many more. It would be very beneficial to have it as a meal about two or three times a week. Don't worry about what people say; copy Jesus (Matthew 14:17–21; Luke 24:41–43; John 21:9–10). Speaking of two or three times a week, you would be remiss to leave the leaves of this tree out of your life. With the exception of the Godhead's *Tree of Life*, the moringa tree has got to be the most significant tree on earth. It may even be the *cousin* of the Tree of Life due to the supreme health benefits and power that comes from it. A branch from the tree does something similar to the event in Exodus 15:23–25. Leaves from the tree are seemingly miraculous in the variety of ways they provide healing.

A little less than six hundred years before the birth of Jesus, the prophet Ezekiel was given a vision by the Lord. Although Ezekiel did not know it, he was describing what will take place in eternity (Ezekiel 47:12). (See the apostle John's description in Revelation 22:2.) In eternity, there will not be a pharmaceutical industry feeding toxic, habit-forming, expensive drugs to the medical institution like some ammunition-carrying soldier feeding ammo into a rapid-firing *mayhem-maker* to pummel the enemy. But leaves from the Tree of Life will be the only all-natural, holistic way the nations will be healed (Revelation 22:2).

In the meantime, here on Earth, it would be in your best interest to start using moringa leaves. A good source where you may obtain them is www.The-Godhead.com.

Essential

Of the thousands of varieties of vegetation the Godhead created to grow from the earth, He infused hundreds with healing power. There are two other substances from the earth that are *must-haves* to complete this chapter: MSM, which is methylsulfonylmethane, and baking soda.

Baking soda, especially the popular Arm & Hammer brand, is ubiquitous here in the US. In contrast to its popularity, however, it appears that people have no idea whatsoever of the myriad ways this superb component of the earth may be used both on and in the body, and for the household. The irony is that people who complain the most about being broke are the ones who waste money on some of the most worthless nonessentials in life. Here are some of the things baking soda may be used for: baking, toothpaste, mouthwash, deodorant, acid indigestion, clogged drains, stain removal, mopping floors, laundry booster, snuffing out small fires, dishwasher, soothing sore muscles, and myriad other uses. Just baking soda alone could replace all the above, and think of how much money you may potentially save in just a year. Hopefully, those who read this will use their common sense to save many cents.

The book I mentioned earlier goes into explicit detail about baking soda and lists about fifty different ways you may use it. When you really think about it, you will avoid all the clutter all the other products would cause. If many across the US did this with baking soda, it could potentially positively impact the nation's landfills. Think about it! Using these natural products daily greatly enhances your DASA mode.

I will close out this chapter with some very revealing information for you to seriously consider. No matter how adamantly allopathic medical physicians and surgeons may deny it, I assert that they use nebulous sophistry in subtly nefarious ways to totally blindside and mentally disarm their patients and win their absolute trust so that patients willingly acquiesce to every sort of bodily mutilation by MDs, not necessarily for the sake of patients' need but for allopaths' financial greed from performing procedures like double

DASA (DYNAMIC APPLICATION OF SPIRITUAL AWARENESS)

mastectomies, ovaries removed, fallopian tubes removed, even full hysterectomies. MDs use their sophistry as scare tactics so that you "voluntarily" accept their suggestions of, "These procedures are *necessary* to decrease the risk of..." or "You need to take this prescription drug for three years to prevent..." or "We can get you started on chemo..." Be aware that much of that is, according solely to an allopathic doctor's opinionated viewpoint, for preventive purposes.

Please pay attention to what some of their own medical peers have always tried to warn patients about, that is,

> Unfortunately, there are more profits to be made in treating disease than in promoting prevention. (Kenneth H. Cooper, MD, MPH)

> We don't know what we're doing in medicine. (Dr. David Eddy)

It just may save your sanity, save your financial integrity, save you from unnecessary surgical mutilation, and even your very life to seek out advice, and/or treatment from a licensed naturopathic doctor (ND) before allowing your precious health to be compromised, your body permanently altered, or your very life *legally* snuffed out by profit-minded allopathic MDs. Speaking of disfiguring one's body, and financial greed, the allopathic medical establishment is partial to, supports, and caters to the frivolous demands of this twentieth-/twenty-first century LGBTQ+ cult that is incongruous to the word of God, as well as brazenly promoting unrighteousness, perversion, and unholiness, not just in the US but worldwide. And with the advocating of hacking off little boy's penises, and little girls' breasts, which allopathic surgeons readily consent to, an unprecedented, heinous level of debauchery and immorality has been reached, a travesty of calamitous proportions.

Lastly, for exceptional, perpetual health, drink an eight-ounce glass of Potent Trio three to five times a day every single day; your body will reward you in more ways than one.

Chapter 10

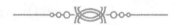

Significance of Christ

For the unbelievers of the world, it is a given that they have no inkling whatsoever of just who Jesus, the Messiah (Christ), really is, who He represents, His profound yet simple teaching and exhortation, and what His purpose was. The mindset of this modern generation is as it was with the Jews two thousand years ago—antagonistic toward Jesus, with sarcastic statements, remarks, and questions: "Where is your father?" "Is he planning to commit suicide?" "Who are you?" "What do you mean, 'You will set us free?'" "You Samaritan devil! Now we know you are possessed by a demon…who do you think you are?" (John 8:19–53).

With so-called advanced knowledge in science and technology, medicine, engineering, and achievements that astound the world (i.e., landing people on the moon), the intellectuals of the world are thought to be enlightened. In truth, however, they are spiritually disfigured and dysfunctional.

Even among those who profess to be Christians, and those who truly are, who show it in their faith in action, still too many have a limited understanding of Christ's significance, who He truly is, and His position in the Godhead. And the only way any saint is going to receive true revelation from Him is to obey Luke 9:23.

I have prayed often and intently that the Holy Spirit empowers me to write effectively, to the point where saints will look at (think about) Jesus with awe and reverence, not with feigned physical emo-

DASA (DYNAMIC APPLICATION OF SPIRITUAL AWARENESS)

tions, but with spiritual exuberance. And once you are fully expressing your dynamic application of spiritual awareness (DASA) in your lifestyle and daily, moment-to-moment actions, you will develop and sustain what Jesus said in John 8:31–32. You will also have the capacity to accept that persecution is part of the bargain (2 Timothy 3:12; 1 Peter 4:12–13).

What I am about to share will surely be refuted by some scholars, Bible teachers, theologians, and pastors. But the Spirit of truth, whose temple is within me, compels me to speak the strict truth.

I am going to start with the first gospel and discuss something that is widely misconstrued among our Christian leaders within varying denominations. Let me first say that there is a clear and distinct difference between *titles* and *names*. Your name identifies who you are, whereas your title shows what you are. Now in your Bible, go on and read Matthew 28:19. Jesus did not command them to baptize people in the titles. He commanded them to do it in the name, not the names but name, which means one name. We are told by 2 Timothy 2:15 to "rightly divide" (correctly explain) God's holy word of truth. And in the book of Acts, you will see that no one was baptized by the titles, but by the name, just one name exclusively. Make no doubt about it, the name of Jesus is all-encompassing, and within that name above all other names is the Father, the Son, and the Holy Spirit (Colossians 2:9). So don't say the titles when you baptize people, say the name (Colossians 3:17).

Who am I? That's not important; it's the One I introduce to you. He's the One you need to know. He's got the answers to all life's mysteries. His name is Jesus; He's the one you need to *really* know, for He is the way (John 14:6).

Pay your utmost attention now, as you are going to meet the One you need to know. The first thing you should know is that there is a holy, harmonious order within the Godhead. However, the context of many leaders' statements potentially leads people to believe that there is a ranking order (i.e., "first Person of the Trinity," "Second Person of the Trinity," and "third Person of the Trinity"). That is nothing more than neologism. And since the entire universe is stamped with the tripartite nature of the Almighty Godhead, I will give you an analogy using something very familiar to you. H_2O, when frozen, is still water; all it does is change composition, but it is still the same water. If you boil it to the point of evaporation, only the composition is changed, but it is still the same water. There is no ranking order between water, ice, and vapor. And that is an example of the tripartite nature the Godhead stamped on the universe, a triune nature. So know this, whether water, ice, or vapor, it is one and the same—H_2O. And whether Father, Son, or Holy Spirit, He is only One—Jesus (John 8:58; 14:7–9; Colossians 2:9).

You might be thinking I am trying to defend Jesus. Not so! After all, who am I? But the Scriptures themselves mightily defend Him. And I am going to back off now and let the sword of the Spirit, the living and powerful word, slash through people's doubts, hesitations, inconsistencies, misconceptions, and incongruities. May the Godhead help you to comprehend and perceive in your spirit just who Jesus is so that you will, in humble reverence, simply say, "Lord, thank You for who You are."

Jesus Himself, as the Word, or "the Word of God" (John 1:1; Revelation 19:13), is indeed the beginning. Case in point:

- Jesus is God's power and wisdom (1 Corinthians 1:24).
- Jesus is God's visible image (John 12:45; Colossians 1:15).
- Jesus is God's secret revealed (Colossians 2:2).
- Jesus is the "container" for God's treasures of wisdom and knowledge (Colossians 2:3).
- Jesus is God's way of making you holy (1 Corinthians 1:2).
- Jesus is the voice of God (Deuteronomy 18:18; Hebrews 1:2).
- Jesus is the Son of God (Luke 1:31–32).
- He is the Son of Man (Matthew 16:13).

Jesus Himself is the Father, not the *essence* of the Father, as some preachers say. He is indeed the Father, just as ice is water. To top it off, Jesus is "the Everlasting Father" (Isaiah 9:6; John 10:30; 8:58). According to Acts 2:36 and 10:36 and Philippians 2:11, Jesus is the one and only Lord. This is certainly supported by other Scriptures.

DASA (DYNAMIC APPLICATION OF SPIRITUAL AWARENESS)

Moreover, in addition to being the One who quenched the Israelites' thirst during their forty-year sojourn in the wilderness (1 Corinthians 10:4), Jesus also is the One who appeared to Moses as alluded to in John 8:58, which may be referenced in Exodus 3:1–14.

There are myriad Scriptures that attest to who Jesus really is, but let's look at just six more:

- Jesus is the Holy Spirit (2 Corinthians 3:17).
- He is the bread of life (John 6:35).
- Jesus is the way, the truth, and the life, as He asserts in John 14:6.
- Jesus gives you the right to become a child of God only by accepting Christ as your Lord and Savior (John 1:12; Romans 10:9).
- Jesus is the light of the world (John 8:12).
- Jesus alone is our High Priest, not the Roman Catholic Pope (Hebrews 4:14).

Lastly, God says He is Lord, and there is no other Savior, as shown in Isaiah 43:11. God also says He is the First and the Last, and there is no other God, no other Rock (Isaiah 44:6,8). Perhaps to an unbeliever, there may appear to be a contradiction between Jesus's claims and God's claims. However, both John and Paul very succinctly provide clarification in John 4:42 as well as Titus 2:13. When you are in DASA mode, the Holy Spirit will enlighten you, bringing you to conclude that the God in Isaiah is none other than Christ Jesus. In fact, Jesus warned everyone that if they refuse to believe His assertive, "I am He" in Deuteronomy 32:39, they will die in their sins (John 8:24, 28). Regarding God saying He is the First and Last in Isaiah 44:6, Jesus gives it even more impact in Revelation 22:12. By this, you should understand clearly the significance of Christ. And keep in mind the significance of the cross (Colossians 1:20–21).

Chapter 11

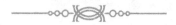

The Gospel Truth

One main reason Christians should invest quality time in both reading and studying the word of God daily is to check the validity of what Christian leaders or Bible teachers are expounding, ensuring it aligns with the truth of the word (Acts 17:11). Most importantly, even if you choose to remain in a specific Christian denomination, do not let it set the precedent for your biblical theology. Let the relevance of Scripture alone guide you as you develop a dynamic application of spiritual awareness.

When the apostle Paul, as a Pharisee, was zealous for his religion, Judaism, that set the precedent for his biblical theology before he came to accept Christ as the Lord of his life (Galatians 1:13–14, 23; Philippians 3:5–6). What we have in this post-modern age are people or groups that selfishly use biblical theology to formulate specific doctrinal systems, for example, African Methodist Episcopal (AME), Apostolic, Baptist, Catholic, Mormon, Reformed, Seventh Day Adventists, and many others. Christendom is replete with divergent denominations. And yes, Judaism is still a major religion mainly for Jewish converts despite what Jesus exhorted and what the apostle Paul wrote extensively about (Matthew 23:15; Philippians 3:7–9).

Acts 4:11–12 is explicit about the name of Jesus, which is corroborated by Philippians 2:9–11, Colossians 2:9 and 3:17. It is faith, the genuine (heartfelt) belief in that name, and confession of your faith in Jesus's name (John 1:12–13; Romans 10:9–10) that enables

DASA (DYNAMIC APPLICATION OF SPIRITUAL AWARENESS)

you to be born into God's kingdom and receive salvation toward eternal life (Matthew 10:38; 1 Peter 1:23). When you add Romans 12:1 to all of this, the Scriptures demand that you be willing to set aside your own personal agenda and be fully devoted to Jesus (Luke 9:23). Continuing in your ways and in "your world" while giving scant time to the Lord is your actions doing the talking, saying, "Sorry, Lord, I'm too busy right now." As the saying goes, "What goes around, comes around." And Luke 17:33 offers a stern warning.

By giving so little time to prayer (actual communication with the Lord) and the lack of personally investing good quality time in the study of the word of God, you leave yourself open to the doctrine of your denomination and the cares of the world, rather than to Jesus (Matthew 13:22). What you need to do is take some *me* time, get to a place where you won't be distracted by anything, not even your smartphone, and seriously examine yourself and your relationship with God; does it line up with the Scriptures? Here are several you may use in a self-assessment:

- Is this really true for you, or is this just religious mysticism (Mark 12:30)?
- Do you believe Jesus is the Father God Almighty? If no, then read these: Isaiah 9:6; John 14:8–9; Colossians 1:15; Hebrews 1:8, 10.
- Are you consistent with what Proverbs 3:9 and Malachi 3:10 say? If you have an excuse for not doing so, read these: Mark 12:43–44; and 2 Corinthians 8:3–5.
- Do you practice any of these: Romans 1:26–27 and Galatians 5:19?
- Do you love Jesus? You're a liar if you continue in your own ways, and you don't obey Him as shown in John 14:21, 23–24 and 1 John 1:6, 3:8.
- Do you live for yourself or for Jesus (2 Corinthians 5:14–15)?

If you profess to be a Christian, and after seriously contemplating those Scriptures you just used to evaluate your Christianity, you discover that you are not the Christian that you should be, then you should realize that you were allowing the spirit of Satan to work in your mind, deceiving you into following his will (Ephesians 2:2; 1 Peter 5:8). And I say this from personal experience. But now, oh how I praise and thank the Lord for pulling me out of the lifestyle of a fake Christian. Now after being strongly chastised by the Lord, I am proud to say I am a Christ-follower and an ambassador for Christ (Psalm 94:12; Proverbs 3:11–12; 1 Corinthians 11:32). I let my light shine brightly now and live for Christ in my thoughts, my words, and my day-to-day, moment-to-moment actions (Colossians 3:17).

Unfortunately, the number of fake Christians in the world today is as countless as sand on the beach. Interestingly, whenever negative repercussions happen based on their own sinful ways, they lay the blame on God (e.g., Judges 21:15). And the "blame-it-on-God" mentality is ubiquitous in today's world.

Even this has a starting point. Guess who started it all? Look no further than your progenitors, Adam and Eve. Adam, wanting to justify himself, pointed the finger back at God, while blaming Eve. Not wanting to be the *fall guy*, she blamed the serpent (Genesis 3:10–13). Who do you shift the blame to for your sins?

So as the Scriptures explicitly show, sin is not God's fault; Satan was the instigator. Satan and his wicked crew of angels who rebelled against God's authority in heaven (Revelation 12:7–9) should be the only ones going to hell according to Jesus (Matthew 25:41; 2 Peter 2:4). God had given a command to Adam, which he undoubtedly shared with Eve (Genesis 2:16–17; 3:2). Then someone else comes and lies to the woman. What she should have done was to consult Adam, and then both of them should have reported the matter to God. But in willful disobedience, they defied God and rejected what He said (Genesis 2:17) in favor of a lie, and to appease their own selfish desire, the very thing that James wrote to warn Christ-followers about in James 1:13–15.

From those times—thousands or millions of years ago, depending on whether you want to believe the word of God or secular science—up until this very day, people (both fake Christians and unbelievers) have thumbed their noses at God by either their words, their

DASA (DYNAMIC APPLICATION OF SPIRITUAL AWARENESS)

actions, or both, and suppress the truth of God by doing what they feel is right for them (Judges 17:6; Romans 1:18, 19, 24–28). Even you, you might be reading these words and saying you are a Christian, and that you go to church, give tithes, and read the Bible. Yet you are "shacking up" with a girl you are not married to (girlfriend, fiancée, friend) because you feel there is nothing wrong with that. That may seem right from a human point of view, but it suppresses God's truth and leads to hell (Proverbs 16:25; 1 Corinthians 6:18–20).

Again, one of the main problems in all of this is the failure of Christ-followers to eagerly and fervently buckle down to make studying the word of God a high priority. Another problem that causes much confusion within the body of Christ (the church) is that one denomination makes a convert "tarry for the Holy Spirit" and "speak in tongues," while another denomination says "tongues will cease, and are no longer in use" (1 Corinthians 13:8). Yet still, another denomination forbids priests to marry and not eat fish on Fridays; other denominations have ministers marrying and eating fish whenever they desire. Some say there will be a *Rapture* of the church, while others say the *Rapture* won't happen until the *judgment day* of the whole world when everyone will rise together to be judged. Also, some denominations baptize by sprinkling a few drops of water on people, while others dunk people in *deep enough* water; some baptize in the titles of "Father, Son, and Holy Spirit," while others do it in the name of Jesus (Matthew 28:19; Acts 2:38). They treat it as a free-for-all!

While all this Scriptural posturing is taking place within Christendom, is it any wonder why the world is left baffled by what to believe and how to come to Christ? The irony is that each Christian denomination believes that they are *in the right* while the other is in error. One denomination, which also forbids females from wearing pants, believes its doctrine is correct; another church believes they are the true church, and that its doctrine of praying to angels (patron saints) and *the Virgin Mary* is correct, and it is apostate to mix in worship or holy communion with any church that is not connected to them. There are denominations that are zealous for the last day of the week (Saturday) as the holy day for worship, believe that your spirit, soul, and body stay in the grave upon death until "judgment day," and they re-enslave people to the law of Moses with their biased doctrine in contrast to what Peter said in Acts 13:38. They twist Scripture like Romans 3:20–22, 25, 28, and 10:4 and Ephesians 2:14–15.

One particular denomination, which does not even refer to itself as Christian, believes that the only name for God is Jehovah, that Jesus is Michael the archangel, that only 144,000 of their group are destined for heaven, that the destiny for the rest of them is a peaceful life here on Earth, and that the Holy Spirit is just a wind, or energetic force that cannot think, see, feel and does not live in believers. Add in the diverse doctrines from the myriad of other denominations, and what we have is a monstrosity—sheer religious chaos!

Despite all the infighting and spiritual disharmony going on between the many religious groups, nearly all of them are prophesying, feeding the poor, visiting incarcerated inmates, caring for orphans, the widows, casting out demons, and many other pious religious activities, whereas some are "working for their salvation." So which of these is the right one? All of them cannot be right. Here is what Jesus says (Matthew 7:21–23 and Luke 18:8). And for any of these thinking they are *it*, here's what Paul says (Romans 3:23).

Moreover, regarding some of these religious denominations, some are just *showboating*, or in it for the money they can rake in from hundreds or even thousands of gullible congregants. To make matters worse, even the church members are attempting to use Proverbs 3:9–10, Malachi 3:10–11, and Luke 6:38 as a cosmic lotto, causing them to become sons of hell (Matthew 23:15).

These are the days Paul was referring to when he wrote to his student, Timothy. And just as people deserted both him and the church back then, it has now far exceeded that (1 Timothy 4:1–5; 6:4–5, 9–10; 2 Timothy 4:10). Just think about it for a while; here we have these diverse denominations all vying for a "position with God." If you are studious in the word of God, these two Scriptures come to mind (1 Corinthians 3:1–9; Hebrews 5:12–14).

Moreover, today's church leaders bicker over which denomination is the greatest like the apostles argued among each other as they

DASA (DYNAMIC APPLICATION OF SPIRITUAL AWARENESS)

were walking to Capernaum about which among them was better. Not having enough of being argumentative, even after Jesus confronted them when they arrived in a house in Capernaum, the apostles were at each other again right in front of Jesus while seated at the "Last Supper" (Mark 9:33–35; Luke 22:24). And that is exactly what is happening between Christian denominations currently.

The question that is probably on the minds of Christians who are not knowledgeable in the Bible is this: "So what will heaven be: an Apostolic heaven, a Baptist one, a Catholic one, a Christian Science one, a Church of God heaven, a Mormon heaven, etc.?" Perhaps unbelievers mockingly think likewise. What's troubling is that many, if not all, Israelis who adhere to Judaism zealously believe they only are children of God by virtue of being born in the lineage of Abraham (compare John 7:47–48 and John 8:33, 39, 41). So many of them still vehemently reject Jesus Christ. Even though it is obvious all through the Old Testament, from Exodus to Malachi, the Jews appear to be oblivious as to why they are scattered throughout the entire world and endure so much antisemitism. All the details may be found in just one chapter of one book—2 Kings 17:1–40. If Judaism were the true religion, then why did Jesus find it a necessary to build His own church as indicated in Matthew 16:18?

Getting back to religious chaos, all the various denominations, some of which have allowed syncretism to creep in, have caused much confusion, complete disunity, infighting, intolerance, and, for the most part, our testimony about Jesus or the word of God is unconvincing to the greater secular world. And God's commands should not be just something we do only on weekends for religious convenience. To be truthful about it, the church, as it currently stands, is in shambles, and I am looking for a mighty move of the Holy Spirit to bring about a spiritual revival that will truly unify us as Jesus said in John 17:21. I pray that a Holy Spirit–empowered, worldwide revival will entice believers to pull away from their TV gods, social media platforms, gaming, smartphone gambling, cards, games, drinking sprees at local bars, Las Vegas, and all the pleasure madness of this secular world, to focus more quality time studying the word of God, and agree on Psalm 19:7–11, and become more involved in the dynamic application of spiritual awareness (Proverbs 22:17; Luke 11:28; James 1:22).

Studying the word of God should not be an option after you come to Christ; it actually is a rite of passage. It is an absolute necessity for spiritual growth and learning how to be an effective representative of Christ. How do you think you will be able to obey Mark 16:15 if "your cup is full of worldliness"? Jesus fills empty cups.

He blesses those who do not see Him but still believe (John 20:29). And He can only "fill your cup" when you extend your hand to Him with your empty cup in it. Notice this:

- The word of God is the spiritual water (John 6:63; 7:38; 1 Peter 1:23).
- Your mind-heart is the empty cup you extend to Jesus (His word, the Bible).
- Then He fills your *cup* with spiritual water, symbolized by you studying the word.

Just as you drink physical water throughout the day every single day for your entire lifetime, you need to drink (study the word of God daily) also from the *water* that is living (Hebrews 4:12), so you will not become spiritually dehydrated. The ninety-nine percent (99 percent) you invest in worldly pursuits in contrast to the one percent (1 percent) you invest in works of the Lord shows your lack of interest in the kingdom of God. You may feel that you are satisfying your desires, wants, and needs by keeping the whole chicken for yourself and giving the Lord just the thin skin. By doing that, however, your attitude is like the men and women who were not satisfied with the Lord (Numbers 11:1, 4–6, 18–20, 32–33). Your worldly lifestyle might seem right to you (Proverbs 16:25). But if you trust God in everything, He will guide you (Proverbs 3:5–6), and also your reward for trusting Him will be the salvation of your soul (1 Peter 1:9). Just that alone is good enough of a reward to delve into DASA with no hesitation. DASA is upward motivation.

Focus intently, and understand that faith in Jesus is the only criterion for salvation. All the subsequent good works you do prove that

DASA (DYNAMIC APPLICATION OF SPIRITUAL AWARENESS)

your faith is genuine (Luke 6:45; 1 Corinthians 15:58); it shows your vested interest in the kingdom of God. Realize this also, those who are in Christ do not acquire only one title; you have multiple titles:

1. child of God (John 1:12)
2. born again (John 3:3)
3. believers (John 20:8; 20:27)
4. saints (Romans 8:27 NKJV)
5. Christians (Acts 11:26)
6. Christ-followers (Luke 9:23)

With the exception of several denominations, nearly all people who have accepted Christ go by one of the above titles. Ironically, I have come across many Catholics who, when asked, "Are you a Christian?" usually respond with, "No, I'm Catholic!" Others will say, "Yes, Baptist!" or "Yes, Seventh-day Adventist!" So many people's answers culminate in naming their denomination. Do they not know that heaven is not compartmentalized (i.e., there are no denominations there)? And much too many people put the intricacies of their denomination above the pure and simple requirements of the gospel. Denominations are man-made and not necessarily 100 percent Christ-centered. Many of them allow too much worldliness or even politics to impact their operation.

The way most people who profess Christianity live their lives, it is as if they willfully ignore:

> Instead, give yourselves completely to God...So use your whole body as an instrument to do what is right for the glory of God. (Romans 6:13 NLT)

This is strongly supported by Romans 12:1–2. God wants us to participate in activities that further His agenda and detach ourselves from worldly ideals (2 Corinthians 6:17). And if you continue to live as the pagans, read James 4:4. There are no games being played here;

God commands you to both repent and to "come out" of that mess (Acts 17:30; Revelation 18:4).

Quite a few people say things like, "I want to enjoy myself while I can," or "You only live once." Believe it or not, multitudes of fake Christians adhere to that secular term. What they lack is knowledge of God's word. Many people think that intense study of the Bible is for ministers of the gospel only. This mindset surely proves Paul's point in 1 Corinthians 3:1–3. Even if you were very sincere when you came to Christ with a humble and remorseful heart, and He saved you because of His mercy and grace, you got off track (Galatians 1:6; 2 Timothy 4:10). That is one of the main reasons we need to drink deeply (study intently) from the word of God every single day while we live here on Earth, and be strong in the Lord and in the power of His might (Ephesians 6:10). Moreover, as I mentioned before, we should be like the people of Berea (Acts 17:11) and make sure by God's word we're not being sucked into denominational doctrine and/or tradition, or syncretism, or sensationalism.

People have varied reasons for making that weekend trek to church. Honestly speaking, all too many men seriously believe they need to be dressed in a suit and tie; and some (a lot) of the women wear high-heel pumps and some outlandish outfits and hats as though they're coming to receive a Hollywood Emmy Award or appearing on Broadway. The issue with that is new converts to Christ, thinking that is the norm, fall into that type of worldliness brought into the church, which is passed down to each successive generation. All of that is nothing but selfishness justified by a lot of poor excuses. Look at what Jesus says in Matthew 16:24–26. And to show you just how ingrained the worldliness is in women, if they knew for a fact that Jesus Christ Himself would be coming to their city the next day at 6:30 p.m., nearly all stores would probably sell out of cosmetics from the hordes of women that would "storm" the aisles looking for the very best makeup to meet Jesus. But that won't happen because He's coming in the blink of an eye, says Paul in 1 Corinthians 15:52. Even Superwoman can't put on her makeup that fast.

Think about it very carefully. Is everything you have or see in this temporary life on Earth worth clinging to and missing all of

DASA (DYNAMIC APPLICATION OF SPIRITUAL AWARENESS)

what Almighty God has in store for you? If you would be so naive as to say, "Yes, because this world has places like Las Vegas, Palm Springs, Beverly Hills, Fifth Avenue, Hollywood, Coach handbags and pumps, Porsches, Bentleys, and so much more." Then your mind is really "out to lunch." You are whacked, a psycho, a lunatic, astonishingly deceived, and devoured (Colossians 2:4; 1 Peter 5:8). All those worldly things rot, fade, and get stolen (Matthew 6:19). To make it worse, all those things are what those on the wide road to hell seek after (Matthew 7:13). Being in DASA mode helps you to transcend such pettiness.

Here are some benefits Christ-followers are going to receive; as a matter of fact, it is so amazing that the Scriptures put it this way:

> Eyes have not seen, nor have ears heard, or
> have come into the imagination of mankind, the
> things God has prepared for those who love Him.
> (1 Corinthians 2:9)

Here is what God offers you:

- Forgiveness of sins: blotted out forever (Isaiah 43:25).
- The right to be God Almighty's own child (John 1:12).
- A new birth: you get to start all over again (John 3:3, 5).
- Eternal life (John 3:36; 17:3).
- No judgment of condemnation (John 5:24; Romans 8:1).
- You receive "living water" (John 7:38).
- You will get a personally prepared suite that is super sweet (John 14:2–3).
- You will have peace in Him (John 14:27).
- Unimaginable joy (John 15:11).
- Untold riches, plus an inheritance (Ephesians 1:14; 3:6; Hebrews 9:15).

You see, when the Lord gives, He gives it *big-time*. And He's just getting started! With what is listed above, that is not even half of it.

So you keep your Bentleys and Hollywood; DASA practitioners will be traversing the universe with the Lord.

After being incessantly bombarded with media of every sort, our minds reach the point of overload. Then it just settles into whatever is trending. Being keen on that, businesses go into high gear, pushing certain popular products toward the trend to the point of *overkill.* And they maximize their profit potential with "keep-it-in-your-face" marketing strategies. That is how they have captured the minds of people to crave cosmetics, and fashion (i.e., name brands, luxury cars, high-powered roadsters, and worldly opulence). They cause people to be mentally enslaved to worldly brand names.

God demands the exact opposite of that (1 John 3:23). Compared to the wealth of knowledge and wisdom in the Godhead (Isaiah 55:8–9; Colossians 2:3), human knowledge and wisdom are that of an embryo attached to an umbilical cord. So rather than allowing our minds and hearts to be enslaved to worldly *brand* names, we should become totally enraptured and captured by *Jesus's* name because He is both God and the Father, as the Scriptures show:

- Jesus is the everlasting Father (Isaiah 9:6).
- Jesus is God (John 1:1, 18).
- Jesus is the Father, the "I AM" (John 8:58).
- Jesus is the Father just as ice is water (John 10:30).
- Jesus is the Father (John 12:45; 14:8–9).
- Jesus is God (Romans 9:5).
- Jesus is God (Philippians 2:6).
- Jesus is the embodiment of the Godhead (Father, Word, Holy Spirit) (Colossians 2:9).
- Jesus is God (Hebrews 1:8; Titus 2:13; 2 Peter 1:1; 1 John 5:20).

Matching Luke 1:35 with Colossians 2:9 will show us that the *incarnation* of Jesus was a process involving the Godhead. And it is Jesus's name that will reverberate across the cosmos (Philippians 2:9–11). That is the gospel truth!

DASA (DYNAMIC APPLICATION OF SPIRITUAL AWARENESS)

As I stated in the first paragraph of this chapter regarding whether someone is preaching, teaching, or speaking the gospel truth, there are three prerequisites to begin to know the difference (John 1:12; 3:3; 8:51):

1. You must believe in Jesus;
2. You must be born again;
3. You must be and stay absolutely committed to, and obey all of the gospel of Jesus Christ.

This is the only way you will be able to get the truth, have the truth, and know the truth. And as you become studious in the word of God, no person, no denomination, no other religion, and no human philosophy will be able to dissuade or cloud your discernment because Jesus, who is truth itself, will liberate you (John 8:31–32, 36; 14:6).

Here is something pertinent you need to understand about repentance. Probably 99.9 percent of new believers in Christ have heard the word *Repent.* "All you have to do is repent!" and not really knowing the truth (John 8:31–32), is easily misled both to and in false teaching because they have never been exposed to the truth. Repentance is not simply to stop doing bad things and to obey the Ten Commandments. It goes much deeper than that. Repentance is all about change; it is about rethinking and reevaluating your lifestyle and then using the word of God to renovate it. This is not taught to new converts, but it should be fully explained before immersion in water (baptism). They should be taught that being baptized in the Spirit (born again), then publicly showing it (water baptism by whole-body immersion), is the beginning of a new way of life (Matthew 4:4; John 6:27; 14:15). And much emphasis should be placed on both Jesus and His gospel of truth. Some points that should be strongly emphasized are:

A. Never be ashamed of the gospel (Romans 1:16).
B. Faith, and only faith in Jesus, is God's way of making you holy; you don't become holy by simply obeying the Ten

Commandments. You show your holiness by allowing the Spirit of God now living inside you to guide your lifestyle (Romans 7:6; Galatians 2:20).

C. Develop a deep desire, hunger, and thirst to study the word of God (Psalm 119:11, 44, 67, 101, 103, 162; Jeremiah 15:16).

D. Keep feeding off the word of God daily so that you may grow spiritually. Teach this to your children, their children, etc. (Psalm 78:5–8).

E. Do not get caught up or entangled in denominational doctrine, nor favor any particular denomination; stay focused on Jesus, the name of Jesus, and the gospel of Jesus (i.e., just be in 24-7 DASA mode).

Lastly, let Jesus be your center and your circumference, stand in awe of, and reverence His holy name. The powerful name of Jesus is the Father's name (John 17:11); the Father sent one of His most elite archangels, Gabriel, to give the young village woman advance notice about the name (Luke 1:31). The Holy Spirit empowered the apostles to baptize new, born again believers in Jesus's name (Acts 2:38). There is no other name in the universe that can save you from hell, except the name of Jesus (Acts 4:11–12). The name of your religious denomination cannot save you, only the magnificent, powerful name of Jesus (Philippians 2:9–11), and that is why your mind, your heart, your mouth, your actions, and your entire lifestyle must be a reflection of Jesus Christ, your Lord, God, Father, High Priest, and Savior (Colossians 3:1). That is the word of Almighty God, and the gospel truth!

Chapter 12

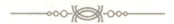

Right Side or Left Side

The terms *apocalypse, Armageddon, end-times, final hour,* and similar expressions have led to much speculation, including wild stories and Hollywood TV shows and movies, causing nothing but confusion, as well as indifference or disbelief in what the word of God indicates as a looming reality. People become very antsy when they must wait a certain amount of time for something, especially if they do not know the exact date of the occurrence.

One of the reasons for people's anxiety is that they rely on their human-based understanding, which is regulated by their emotions. These emotions are in a constant state of flux, being directed by varying unforeseen circumstances. Additionally, people are enslaved to time and are unable to comprehend phenomena outside of that realm. For this reason, they become indifferent and oblivious to the biblical meaning of the word *soon* (e.g., when Jesus Himself says, "I am coming soon!" (Revelation 22:7, 12, 20). Therein lies the problem; humans take a spiritually relayed word and desire to place it in a finite time realm. It also shows they do not know the Scriptures, which answer how soon (Matthew 24:36; Acts 1:7; 1 Thessalonians 5:1–2).

No one can humanly relate to spiritual truth, and that is why people relegate the parables of Jesus to the same box containing the Easter Bunny, Saint Patrick's Day, and Santa Claus Day. It is downright demeaning to the holy name of Jesus to associate Christ with

December 25, and I dare not call that day Christmas. I call it "Santa's Day" because he is the god nearly the whole world worships annually and teaches that ungodly day to children. Christians try hard to justify celebrating Easter by saying the egg represents the stone that was rolled away from the grave tomb of Jesus. I guess there were bunnies hopping quickly away also. So-called Christmas has as many justifications as "needles" on their pine tree, which, somehow, morphs into a "Christmas tree" once a year. Rather than celebrate two wholly holy events (the Sabbath and the Passover) pertaining to God Almighty as indicated in Genesis 2:3, Isaiah 58:13, Deuteronomy 16:1, and Acts 20:16, children of God ignore Romans 12:2, James 4:4, and 1 John 2:15–16 and participate with unbelievers of the world in celebrating the "Easter" bunny and Santa's Day. There will be a price to pay for church leaders who take part in and support that syncretism (1 Corinthians 3:12–15).

One particular parable of Jesus talks about separating sheep on His right side and goats on His left. People pass this off as just another of the hundreds of familiar stories read as children: *Paul Bunyan, Goldilocks and the Three Bears, Peter Pan, Cinderella, Humpty Dumpty*, etc. Contrarily, all of Jesus's parables are connected to a forthcoming reality and an urgent warning, with many of them alluding to or directly speaking of Judgment Day, which only those who ignore and reject the gospel of Christ will face (Isaiah 66:15–16; 2 Thessalonians 1:8).

Caught

With the multitude of church splits, numerous denominations, and syncretism, confusion, misquotes, and misconceptions have spread like wildfire throughout Christendom. One main event I want to clear up here is the liberation of Christ-followers from this sin-infested world. Above all else, make sure you use a DASA branding iron to seal in your mind what I am about to share with you. And do not, under any circumstances whatsoever, allow any denomination to dilute, pollute, confute, or steal this truth and solid proof

DASA (DYNAMIC APPLICATION OF SPIRITUAL AWARENESS)

from you. Are you ready? Okay, here it is—Luke 9:23 believers will not face judgment:

- John 3:18; 5:24
- Romans 5:9; 8:1
- 1 Corinthians 11:31–32; 1 Thessalonians 1:10; 5:9

When you accept Jesus as your Lord according to Romans 10:9–10, and God knows whether you are serious or just acting on your emotions, at that moment you become *born again*. Listen carefully, DASA practitioners. You were reborn with living water (John 7:39) who carries the word of God (Ephesians 6:17), and you will live forever in Christ (1 John 2:23).

With that stated, let me also share this with you. When the Lord Jesus returns to judge the world, you will not be here. How so? Because you will be following behind Jesus when He comes (1 Corinthians 6:2; Jude 14–15). You want to know how you got there? It was via 1 Thessalonians 4:14–17 because it happens about seven years before the judgment day of Matthew 24:30–31. Christ will descend from the sky and actually come down to earth as other Scriptures connected to Matthew's passage will show. Since saints will not be included in the judgment, they must be snatched (caught up) out of this world, as 1 Thessalonians 4:14–17 clearly shows. For even more details on it, see 1 Corinthians 15:35–57. This is not the same as the judgment.

The Judgment

In three of the four Gospels, Jesus used numerous parables, illustrations, and analogies to depict Judgment Day (Armageddon; D-Day). Let's examine some of them to let you know how deadly serious Jesus was. And all He was doing was sharing and explaining precisely what was to come. There is not one single conjecture, fabrication, or lie in any of this because it is impossible for God to lie (Hebrews 6:18), and Jesus is God.

Starting with Matthew 8:12, it shows people being tossed into not just darkness but outer darkness. Two other leaders made it sound like the gloomiest of doom (2 Peter 2:17; Jude 1:13). I don't even want to try to imagine what that's going to be like. And they are going to weep and grit their teeth from some type of agony. Moving on to Matthew 13:42. It shows why people will be weeping and gritting their teeth in sheer agony. By saying, "That is the way it will be at the end of the world," verse 50 supports the above statement. Matthew 22:13 provides another parable for the same event, while Matthew 24:30 sheds a little more information about it.

Now Matthew 25:30–46, still discussing the same event, delves into more detail. It describes Jesus sitting on His throne to pass judgment, separating those who, in their shame and humiliation, accepted Jesus as Lord and Savior during the seven-year tribulation period, to His right side (the sheep), from those who chose to continue in sins and refused to accept Christ, on His left (the goats). Remember, the *church* (a.k.a. body of Christ; born again believers, Christ-followers, saints, Christians) will be caught up out of this world seven years before Judgment Day. After being caught up, many of those left behind will, at some point during the seven years prior to Jesus's final return, come to their senses (the sheep).

In Dr. Luke's Gospel, he gives us a slightly different perspective on the same Judgment Day scenario (Luke 13:28–30). Did you notice that those unbelievers in torture (verse 28) will be able to see the saints "chillin' out" with Jesus, who will share a meal with His saints, pick fruit from the Tree of Life and give them some, and even let saints sit on His unbelievably awesome throne (Revelation 2:7; 3:20–21)? I assume the way judged unbelievers and rejecters of Christ will be able to see it will be somewhat similar to the rich man in Luke 16:23–26. Moving on a few chapters to Luke 21:25–28, he shares with us the sheer terror people at the end of the seven-year tribulation period will feel when they actually see the One they neglected gliding down from heaven in power, glory, and with the uncountable angels and saints trailing behind. Perhaps we can call this the flying, holy retinue. However, the ones still living who came to their senses during the seven-year period will not be in ter-

DASA (DYNAMIC APPLICATION OF SPIRITUAL AWARENESS)

ror according to verse 28. For all who are killed for accepting Christ in their hearts during those godless seven years, Revelation 7:13–14 provides details on them.

Revelation 1:7 encapsulates Christ's final return. Let's reverse directions now and examine another slightly different explanation of what will happen to the judged people; I call them the living dead, spiritual zombies (2 Thessalonians 1:8–9). It is really unfortunate that so many will choose to burn rather than accept the generous, loving offer of Jesus (Matthew 7:13). Even seven hundred years before the Word became human, one particular prophet stated the "Grave is licking its lips" in anticipation of all the billions of men and women who will be, and already are, on that wide road (Isaiah 5:14 NLT). So many people lean on the false assumption that a loving God would not condemn people to death. Well, you are the one condemning yourself; He does not want you to perish, according to 2 Peter 3:9.

Nevertheless, as Creator, Almighty God reserves the exclusive right to both create and/or destroy life:

I am the One who kills and gives life. (Deuteronomy 32:39)

The Lord gives both death and life. (1 Samuel 2:6)

Fear only God, who can destroy both body and soul in hell. (Matthew 10:28).

Repent, or God will tear you apart. (Psalm 50:22)

Jesus holds the keys to death and the grave. (Revelation 1:18)

There are two types of breath that the Lord will give:

1. the breath of eternal life (John 7:39; 20:22), or

2. or the breath of death, separating you from the presence of God for eternity (Isaiah 11:4; 30:28, 33; and 2 Thessalonians 2:8–9).

That last one is a *holy inferno*!

The choice is yours, and only yours to make. Make a wise choice; choose the name above all other names—Jesus (Philippians 2:9)!

Chapter 13

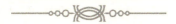

The End-Times

In other chapters, we covered various aspects of the end of this current life as we know it. However, this chapter covers it in explicit detail as showcased in the book of Revelation. We commence by highlighting the birth, death, and resurrection of Jesus, leading us to His climactic second return, which results in a new beginning.

First coming of Jesus: It is important, as a practitioner of DASA, to thoroughly understand how the sword of the Holy Spirit makes it explicit to Christ-followers about this twofold occurrence:

1. Birth/death: Jesus was born in a mortal body that was viewed by the world (Isaiah 9:6; Luke 2:5–20; John 19:28–30); both believers and unbelievers saw Him, and He died in a mortal body.
2. Resurrection: Jesus was raised in a body of immortality but made Himself visible only to Christ-followers; the unrepentant world could not see Him (Mark 16:1–6; Luke 24:35–43; 1 Corinthians 15:3–8).

Second coming of Jesus: Now bear in mind that just as His first coming was a twofold occurrence, likewise for the forthcoming event; however, it will be the reverse of His first coming. When He came into the world and was subsequently killed, all eyes viewed it, including His burial. But after His resurrection, Jesus was invisible to the world of unbelievers and those who disregarded Him.

1. Appearance: Jesus will come down from heaven accompanied by all Christ-followers who died at any time prior to this occurrence, whether it was fifteen minutes ago or two thousand years ago. However, He will not land on Earth; instead, He will appear in the clouds, and with the powerful shout of His word, call saints up there to meet Him. This event will be invisible to the unrepentant world (1 Thessalonians 4:14–17). For a bit more detail, see 1 Corinthians 15:35, 40, 42–44, and 50–54.

2. Appearance: With an entourage of "caught up" Christ-followers and the armies of heaven (angels) trailing Him, Jesus descends to Earth magnificently and majestically on a white horse. The eyes of Jesus will be ablaze like inferno flames, and when His feet make touchdown atop the Mount of Olives, there will be a sonic boom that will split it in half, north to south (Zechariah 14:4–9; Luke 21:25–27; Revelation 1:7; 19:11).

This event, which happens about seven years after His dramatic but invisible air show experienced only by saints, will be visible to every eye on planet Earth, as the Scriptures show. The seven-year period between His twofold second coming is called *the great tribulation*, which itself is a two-fold occurrence of three and one-half years (forty-two months, or a time, times, and half a time) each. Jesus's final, visible return at the end of the tribulation is necessary to prevent mankind from total self-destruction (Mark 13:20), while simultaneously establishing His everlasting kingdom on Earth (Revelation 11:15).

Understand this: The Bible (the sword of the [Holy] Spirit, Ephesians 6:17) is not a book full of contradictions, as ignorant haters of Jesus will try to make you believe. Rather, it is the most organized, thought-out, comprehensive unit of spiritual literature in existence, consisting of a total of sixty-six books that help individuals seeking God, with a sincere heart, to *find* Him (1 Chronicles 28:9).

DASA (DYNAMIC APPLICATION OF SPIRITUAL AWARENESS)

I challenge you to read each of the following Scriptures from Genesis to Revelation and see if you find any contradiction or inaccuracy: Genesis 6:5, Judges 21:25, Nehemiah 9:26–29, Romans 6:23, Galatians 6:8, Titus 1:16, 2 Peter 2:4, Revelation 9:20. What you will find in those Scriptures, however, are warnings. As you know, there are reasons for warnings: to help prevent you from destruction. And the Godhead would really prefer everyone to be saved (Romans 2:4; 1 Timothy 2:4; 2 Peter 3:9).

It is really sad that there will nevertheless be obstinate people who choose not to have a life of eternal peace in the presence of God but would rather stay on the wide road to hell, as Jesus plainly stated (Matthew 7:13). And believe it or not, there will be both Jews and Gentiles choosing that way, many! Only a remnant (few) of both groups will choose Matthew 7:14 and 22:37, Luke 9:23, and Romans 6:12–13. That remnant of Jews saved is God's love for them, as well as keeping the promise He made regarding them (Isaiah 65:9; Zechariah 8:11–12; Matthew 8:11–12). The so-called *replacement theology*, though it is having a negative effect on some Christian leaders and believers, still will not negate the truth of God's holy word. And here is the truth: both Jews and Gentiles are united as one church in Christ (1 Corinthians 12:27; Galatians 3:26–29; also see Ephesians 2:15–16, 19–22). The explicitness in 1 Corinthians 12:13 reveals the consensus of the Godhead in removing the distinction between Jew and Gentile, making them all one in Christ, sealed by His blood. This is emphasized in Galatians 3:28.

Seeing Jesus striding through space down to the holy city of Jerusalem and setting up His headquarters there, Satan snatches out his contact list, hooks up with his two "yes-men" (the beast and false prophet), and ramps things up by sending their demon agents to all their contacts of world leaders to stage a coup against Jesus and company (Revelation 16:13, 14, 16).

Allow me to interject something here to help you avoid becoming confused as these scenes play out. Revelation is not in chronological order. So you need to know that the following Scriptures are simply different descriptions of the exact same event, which, when combined, show the tripartite action of the Godhead:

- seals—Revelation 6:12–17 (seals of Jesus)
- trumpets—Revelation 8:7–12; 9:1–21 (trumpets of God)
- bowls—Revelation 16:1–21 (bowls of the Holy Spirit)

The attempted coup backfired (Revelation 17:14), and with all the 1 Thessalonians 4:14–17 saints with Him, Jesus defeated His enemies with the sharp "sword of the Lord" that flew from His mouth, making fresh meat dumplings out of the millions of attackers. The beast and the false prophet were captured and, bypassing hell, those two were tossed directly into the worst of the worst (Revelation 19:15, 20). And one of the angels, who could speak bird language, rallied the sky-high, circling vultures—probably thousands of them—and invited them to a "human dumpling feast" (Revelation 19:17–18, 21). As for the beast's and false prophet's boss, bad boy Satan was manhandled by a big, burly, planet-wrestling angel who chained him up, then threw him into a pit with no bottom to it for a thousand years, as shown in Revelation 20:1–3.

Finally, with the earthshaking, universe-rattling, fiery wrath of God subsided, two Scriptures come true (Luke 2:14 and also 1 Corinthians 6:2). And all the saints who died in the aftermath of the seven-year tribulation period, who came to life again (Revelation 20:4), are the ones Revelation 7:9–16 mentions. This is the one-thousand-year peace period where saints will be given authority to both judge and serve as holy priests, as Peter spoke of (1 Peter 2:9; Revelation 20:5), described by another prophet in Isaiah 65:17–25. Unfortunately, there is one more disturbance that must take place that the Scriptures be fulfilled, and saints will enjoy truly eternal peace afterward, a peace prophesied in 2 Peter 3:13.

During both the seven-year tribulation and the one thousand years of peace, people will still die from natural causes, accidents, or some other cause. The final disturbance that takes place is what the Godhead uses to test the validity of people's hearts and their faith, as He has always done (Genesis 22:1; Job 7:18; Proverbs 17:3; James 1:3). There are people who, no matter how much respect, kindness, patience, compassion, and love you extend to them, show no appreciation, are perpetually evil, and with depravity of heart and mind,

DASA (DYNAMIC APPLICATION OF SPIRITUAL AWARENESS)

choose Satan over Jesus. So the Lord will release the devil to test the true intentions of all to see who loves Christ according to Matthew 22:37, Luke 14:28, and John 14:15. And the weeds are rooted out according to Matthew 3:12 and 13:27–30. It is those *weeds* that join Satan upon his release from his one-thousand-year sentence, and they attempt to bum-rush and obliterate Jesus, the saints, and the Lord's holy Jerusalem headquarters (Revelation 20:7–8). Satan does this alone because his two losers are unable to assist him.

Jesus looks at this last-ditch effort by His nemesis somewhat like a gnat or fly that needs to be swatted. He did not even waste His time or energy allowing the armies of heaven to battle this innumerable mass of attackers spread out on the plains beyond Jerusalem as far as the eyes could see. So showing everyone that He is supremely the one and only King of all kings and Lord of all lords (Revelation 17:14 and 19:16), Jesus, hardly even lifting a finger, performed the "Elijah move" (2 Kings 1:10) and roasted the entire army like campfire marshmallows, with a single puff from heaven (Revelation 20:9). Then the beast and the false prophet, who by now have been torturously sizzling like French fries in superhot grease for those ten hundred years, received some company; bad boy Satan, who has always been sizzling mad at Jesus, will now be sizzling for all eternity (Revelation 20:10). Checkmate!

So if you do not want to face God Almighty in the wrath of His fiery, flaming judgment on disobedient children of God, and on those who do not know God (2 Thessalonians 1:8–9), then consider the dynamic application of spiritual awareness (DASA). Learn it, breathe it, practice it daily, get fully engaged in it, make it your lifestyle, become proficient enough to effectively demonstrate it and correctly teach it one-on-one or to a group.

Become DASA-minded and stay in (reside in) DASA mode until you are in the presence of the Lord, who will welcome you to the brand-new wholly holy heavens and earth He creates, where there will be no need for an ocean nor lights because heavenly H_2O will flow directly from His throne, and the Godhead will be the only source of light (Revelation 21:1–4, 23; 22:1–2). Moreover, no more remembrance of this life will come to mind (Isaiah 65:17).

Conclusion

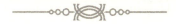

The Word (John 1:1) simply spoke, and all the planets and stars appeared from nothing to form the magnificent cosmos, the entire universe (Psalm 33:9 and 148:5; 2 Peter 3:5).

That unimaginably powerful word is the dynamic force currently sustaining the entirety of the Word's creation, as shown in Hebrews 1:3. Not surprisingly, the Word's word is the very foundation upon which DASA is built, and DASA is empowered by the Holy Spirit.

Now consider this: ever since the Word spoke creation into existence, there has been continuous, unceasing (dynamic) motion: shining stars, spinning planets, planets revolving around the sun. Never, ever has this movement ceased, with the exception of one particular event where the Lord halted Earth's rotational spin for a few hours (Joshua 10:12–14).

With that in mind, you must realize it is the living word of God (Hebrews 4:12) that hones your dynamic application of spiritual awareness, as the Holy Spirit Himself works within you, churning your DASA so that you will not become stagnant, nor will you tire from doing good works (Galatians 6:9; 2 Thessalonians 3:13). Moreover, serve the Lord joyfully and with faithful enthusiasm. Nothing you do for Him is useless. There are benefits (Proverbs 19:17; Matthew 6:33; 1 Corinthians 15:58). DASA, in and of itself, is nothing but an empty shell, a useless concept without the word of God. Therefore, invest as much time as possible in studying the word.

As a honed DASA practitioner, unaffected by or unfazed by human emotions, you dwell in the triune nature of the Godhead:

- He is holy (Revelation 4:8). The character, essence, and substance of the Godhead are wholly holy. Saints are drenched in the holiness of Jesus, which drives out sin.
- He is light (1 John 1:5). Light cannot be defeated by darkness; light completely overcomes darkness. Saints are children of Light (1 Thessalonians 5:5).
- He is love (1 John 4:8). The agape love of the Godhead conquers hate. Saints who love their enemies do not respond to the physical emotion of hate (Matthew 5:44–48).

Being in DASA mode 24-7 keeps you mindful of both who and what you are; you are the light of the world (Matthew 5:14). And your light should shine perpetually (Philippians 2:15). The heavenly presence that is within DASA practitioners surpasses all human understanding and goes beyond any human logic that is known:

1. The Spirit of the Father (1 Corinthians 3:16)
2. The Holy Spirit (1 Corinthians 6:19)
3. The Spirit of Christ (Galatians 4:6) dwells in saints, not for you to do and live as you please, but to help you help Him to help you help Him carry out His own purpose.

So keep breathing the DASA way to stay in DASA mode until His appearance (1 Thessalonians 4:14–18; also see 1 John 3:2).

I leave you with this profound statement: The entire word of God (the Holy Bible) is a reflection of His tripartite nature. From Genesis to Malachi represents the Father, the four Gospels represent Jesus, and Acts through Revelation represents the Holy Spirit. Cogitate on that. Shalom!

About the Author

Adym Dantz, formerly a superficial Christian, came to his senses during his prison incarceration. During this period, the author sensed a strong conviction from the Holy Spirit. He started not just reading but intently studying the word of God to the point of being studious, often engaging in all-night vigils. Eventually, the author became a Luke 9:23 Christ-follower, and through God's promises, he received a triple blessing: spiritually, physically, and financially. Realizing he is the temple of the Almighty, holy Godhead (1 Corinthians 3:16, 6:19 and 2 Corinthians 13:5), Adym relinquished his all to the Lord as commanded in Romans 12:1–2 and is able to be in DASA mode perpetually in deference to Colossians 3:16–17.

www.ingramcontent.com/pod-product-compliance
Lightning Source LLC
LaVergne TN
LVHW041612131224
799068LV00001B/60